WHAT SHOULD I FEED MY Baby?

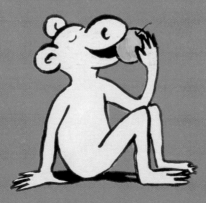

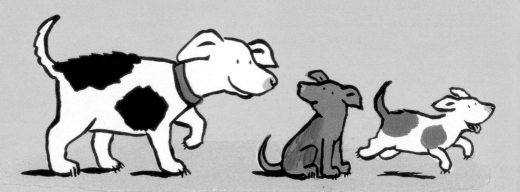

WHAT SHOULD I FEED MY *Baby?*

THE COMPLETE NUTRITION GUIDE FROM BIRTH TO TWO YEARS

SUZANNAH OLIVIER

RECIPES BY SUSAN HERRMANN LOOMIS

ILLUSTRATIONS BY EMILY BOLAM

WEIDENFELD & NICOLSON

TO MY SON, BENEDICT

Please note that none of the information in this book is
intended as an alternative to medical advice, which you must
seek if concerned about your child.

I have elected to use the male gender throughout the book
for ease – with apologies to parents of little girls!

Text Copyright © 1998 by Suzannah Olivier

Suzannah Olivier has asserted her moral right to be identified
as the author of this book in accordance with the Copyright,
Design and Patents Act 1988.

Illustrations Copyright © 1998 Emily Bolam
Design Copyright © 1998 Weidenfeld & Nicolson

First published in 1998 by Weidenfeld & Nicolson

This edition first published in 2003 by Weidenfeld & Nicolson

The Orion Publishing Group
Orion House
5 Upper St. Martin's Lane
London WC2H 9EA

British Library Cataloguing-in-Publication Data
A catalogue record for this book is available from the British
Library.

ISBN 0-297-84354-0

Designed by Nigel Soper

Printed and bound in Italy by Printer Trento S.r.l.

CONTENTS

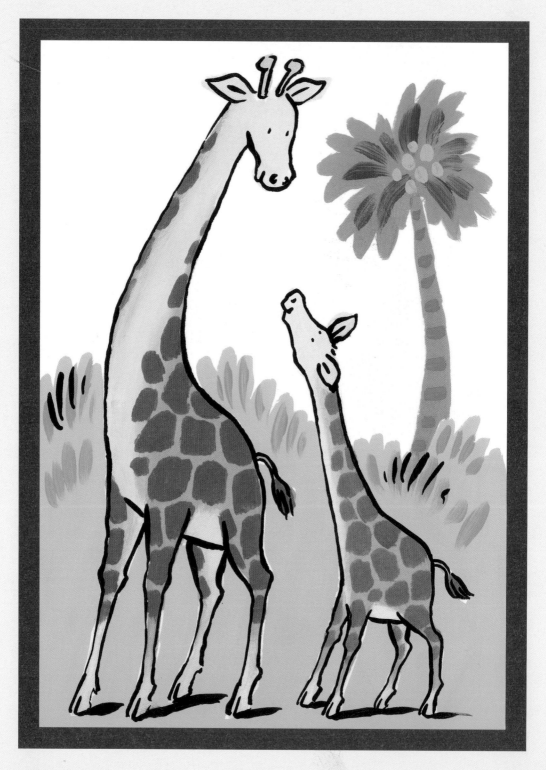

WHY DO YOU
AND YOUR CHILD
NEED THIS BOOK?

YOU HAVE A WONDERFUL, new, little being, who is totally dependent on you and the decisions you make for his welfare. Nutritionally speaking, he is a blank slate and you have the opportunity to provide the best building materials and fuel for him to grow, develop and thrive.

You will, almost inevitably, be faced with a barrage of information, advertising and personal stories related to nurturing your child – much of it conflicting. Many people know more about the running of their computer or their car than they do about the running of their bodies. We need an instruction manual. If I had my way, nutrition would be taught in all schools – it is the basis of health, good or poor, from the womb to the tomb. Sadly, the subject is not taught in schools, nor is it taught in most medical schools.

Each day we put food into our mouths, and into the mouths of our children, without knowing what effect it may have and what the best options are. In this book I hope to give you the principles that will help to ensure your child has the best opportunity, from a nutritional standpoint, to grow into a happy and healthy adult.

The nutritionist in me aims to give you the best and most current information that is available to help you raise a healthy, happy child – and this book is dedicated to that aim. The working parent in me, however, realizes that the ideal must be tempered by the reality of busy lives and existing entrenched habits. Even the most informed parents often have excellent intentions but limited time.

This is not a book of rules, but a guide providing all the necessary information to enable you to find your own way. It is here for reference and, in particular, the meal-planner sections will give you a good idea of how to put all the information together. What I do not want is to create anxiety about the need to get it right all the time. Opinions and choices relating to food are endless and it can be a confusing minefield. Choose what you feel is appropriate in this book for you and your child – you know more about what is right for your lifestyle than any "expert" dictating the ideal situation.

Enjoy this book and enjoy putting the relevant parts, for you, into practice. Discover the possibilities of different foods and different cuisines that will give your child the best possible start in life – and most of all, enjoy your child!

Suzannah Olivier

CHANGING
HABITS

Whataever putting together a dietary plan for your baby, it will soon become clear that you will need to address the eating habits of the whole family. If not, the groundwork that you so carefully lay down may slip as soon as your baby starts to eat meals with the grown-ups.

Changing habits is often not easy, because they are just that – habits. It may be that your diet is already a healthy one, in which case adding a few more positive points should be reasonably easy. Possibly you have flicked through this book already and have blanched at the list of measures for giving your child the ideal diet. Alternatively, you may be so inspired by the measures that you have already written down a long list of dos and don'ts and a shopping list several pages long.

Many of us have high expectations about a new approach to some aspect of our lives – be it a diet, a new exercise regime, getting up earlier, doing more work or whatever – only to be disappointed. And yet, if approached in a way that works for you, the transition can be almost painless. The trick is…

EASY DOES IT

I know people who, in a bustle of enthusiasm, have gone out and spent a fortune on new foods, only to find a few weeks later that their live yoghurts are growing mould in the fridge, their oatcakes are soggy and packets of seeds have gone stale. The reason is that, during the hurry of their day, they have skipped the new regime and turned to their usual staples.

When I advise people on their diets, I prefer to give them a few clear, easy measures that they can incorporate without disrupting their whole lives. A few weeks later we will go to the next stage. The process of changing their diet can take months, or longer. The advantage of going the slow route is that the changes tend to be forever instead of for a few weeks.

If you are reading this book before your baby is born or just after the birth, you have around nine months before he is able to eat some of the same meals as the rest of the family, so you have plenty of time. If it is later than this, it is never too late – you and your baby or toddler will always benefit. Nor is it too late if you have already pursued a different approach with an earlier child – you can use this information just as readily.

I have found that good dietary habits are best founded on what you are already doing that is right – just do more of it, more often. So if, for instance, you like eating fish but only do so once a week, make it twice a week. If you like fruit but only have a couple of pieces a day, edge it up to three or even four pieces a day and buy a wider variety of produce. If lentils are a favourite but do not feature on the menu often then here is a reminder.

THE TIMES ARE A-CHANGING

When I first wrote this book, some of the concepts it explained, such as how to improve on formula milk, reduce colic and avoid food sensitivities, were quite daring and took the cutting edge approach of Optimum Nutrition. However, now these measures are moving into the mainstream.

Formulations for infant milks are a good example. Obviously we all know that breast is best and I would always encourage any mother to breast feed for as long as she is able. But the reality is that most mothers who breast feed give up after six or twelve weeks. Maybe this is to do with modern life and how we are all so busy?

But if you turn to formula milks, the idea that you might be able to improve on them in the simplest possible ways, was pretty radical when I first suggested it. Well, now we are slowly seeing the very improvements I was talking about a few short years ago creeping into infant formulas. Very important essential fatty acids and LCPs (long chain polyunsaturated fatty acids) vital for brain and eye health are now being included in the formulations of some milks by forward thinking companies, who are market leaders, based on expert research.

The idea that you can improve a baby's digestive comfort (colic) and bowel movements by adding prebiotics and probiotic (beneficial bacteria) ingredients to drinks is no longer strange and prebiotics, which encourage a healthy digestive tract are being added to at least one leading formula milk.

Being aware of food sensitivities in a baby is now more commonplace and is a practice that can allow a baby to grow up being more free of a whole range of common modern infant health problems such as glue ear and eczema.

This is all very satisfying! But what is not improving is the overall diet of children on a typical Western diet – and yet this is relatively easy for a caring parent to remedy. Bringing up a nutritionally healthy baby is not a complicated event. Good food, a variety of taste sensations, a family that eats together with reasonable regularity, and a large dollop of love is all that is needed. It also helps to know some of the nutritional basics and to have a little inspiration on tap, both of which many mothers have told me this book provides for them.

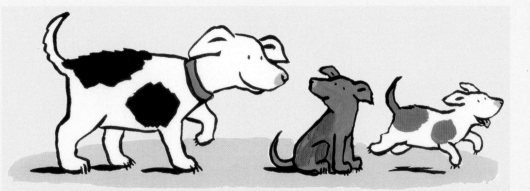

HEALTHY
CHILDREN MAKE
HEALTHY ADULTS

Diet is intimately related to health. Your baby is the sum of all the food that you, the mother, ate during pregnancy, and what he has subsequently eaten and digested – nothing more and nothing less. So the quality of that food, and the ability to digest it properly, determines the nature of your child's cells and body processes – after taking genetics into account. All foods are not equal and you can dramatically help your child to optimum health with good food choices.

There is mounting evidence that the basis of good health in adult years is laid down in a child's formative years:

❦ A child born with a good sized (but not an enlarged) liver, where cholesterol is metabolized, has a lower risk of cardiovascular disease in later life.

❦ Children as young as 10, on poor diets, are showing early stages of "furring up" of arteries.

❦ Teenage girls with high salt and low potassium diets (junk food) are showing early stages of osteoporosis. Also suspected is the high phosphoric acid intakes from the carbonated drinks that so many children consume.

❦ Studies show that when there is obesity in childhood, there is an 80% chance for this to be the case in adulthood.

You do not need to be concerned, however, that you may have done harm if your diet was less than perfect during pregnancy – Mother Nature can be very forgiving. Every cell, and indeed every molecule, in the human body renews itself in six to twelve months in small children. Therefore the potential to replace, repair and create good health is fantastic if we provide the right raw materials.

PREVENTION IS BETTER THAN CURE

There are early warning signs for what I shall call 'reduced health'. This is not necessarily overt disease, or clinical symptoms that your doctor would identify, but just being below par.

In a child this might appear as crankiness for long periods of time, dark circles under the eyes, regular digestive upsets, rough skin, listlessness or overexcitability. Unfortunately, a small child cannot communicate verbally so parents have to be vigilant. This does not mean being neurotic about the smallest change, but monitoring health over a period of time to get a picture of what is normal for your child and what may require attention.

My experience is that if you are alert to, and deal with, 'reduced health' in your child, you can prevent many of the more serious childhood problems from developing. For instance, if you have a child who tends towards food sensitivities, pay attention to occasional diarrhoea and constipation, nappy rashes or 'allergy circles' around his eyes, and you may avoid having a child who develops uncomfortable eczema or headaches.

The main killers – heart disease, cancer and diabetes – have a strong genetic link. We are often told to expect the worst if the disease is in the family. But these diseases are also largely related to dietary habits, a fact substantiated by the United States Surgeon-General and by the World Health Organization. Diet can be as "hereditary" as genes.

As important as preventing disease, however, is giving the optimum start in life to your child, so that he will flourish to meet his full potential and grow to be a happy, healthy adult.

WHAT IS OPTIMUM NUTRITION?

Concerned parents will know that there are nutritional guidelines that have been set up to rear the average healthy child. But your child is not average – she or he is a unique little being. What is right for one child may not be right for another. You want the best for your child as an individual. The optimum for your child will be different to that for another.

There are three basic concepts that are fundamental to optimum nutrition:

Every individual is unique: So much advice is given for the 'average' child, and yet do you know an average child? Genetic factors will determine the different reactions that children will have to foods and nutrients. Foods will be digested, absorbed and utilized differently from one child to another. Different genetic factors will also determine individual needs for specific nutrients. One child will need, for example, more fats in his diet and another more proteins; yet another will need more zinc or vitamin C than the 'average' child.

No one nutrient works alone: We live in a time of fashion trends when particular foods or nutrients will suddenly become the buzz of the moment. Lately, for instance, guidelines have been given that all mothers should, quite rightly, take 400 mcg of folic acid preconceptually and throughout the first trimester to help reduce the risk of neural tube defects. Some mothers may be given iron for anaemia in the last trimester. Parents are urged to ensure their children get 500 mg of calcium a day.

And yet nutrients do not come in isolation in food or in nature. They come with a broad range of co-factors with which they work, and which ensure that they work optimally. Folic acid works with B12 and vitamin C helps its usage. Anaemia may not be due to just iron deficiency, but to low levels of zinc, which helps the usage of iron, or even to insufficient essential fats, which help to bind the iron. Calcium works best with magnesium and vitamin D. This may all sound complicated but so is the human body! Luckily, good foods are wiser than physicians and provide a whole array of nutrients.

Environmental factors affect each individual differently: The child living in a city centre will have different needs to the child who lives by the sea. The stress levels that the child is exposed to will make a difference nutritionally. Even the type of food that a child is given is an environmental concern since all food is part of the environment – or an outside influence – until assimilated into the body. So foods that have chemical residues or preservatives will impact on a child's body differently to foods that are free of these substances.

Taking these principles into account, I hope to give you the power to make the best decisions for your child in relation to his or her diet. I would also like to give you the ability to sort through the conflicting advice that you will encounter all the time, including advertising pressure, and decide if the information you are receiving makes sense or not.

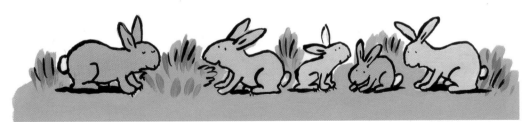

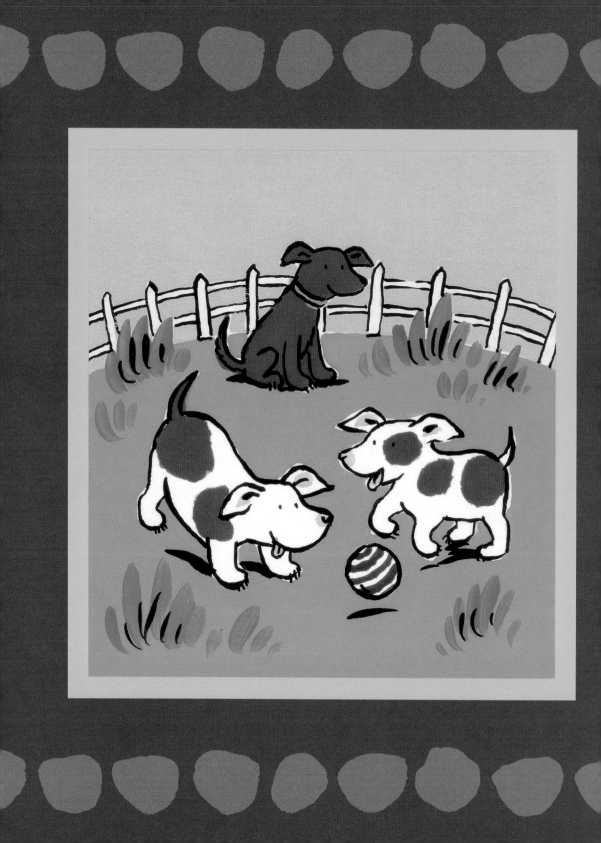

1

WHAT ARE LITTLE CHILDREN MADE OF?

Little boys and little girls are made of water, proteins, fats, minerals and small stores of carbohydrates and vitamins – the quantities in that order. Little boys and little girls are actually the most wonderfully complex soup of chemical reactions that Mother Nature has been able to dream up, with that extra-special something that makes them the unique individuals you love so much.

THE FIRST
YEAR OF PHYSICAL
GROWTH

You do not have to study science to be astounded by the amazing development of one fertilized egg into a complete little human being. Buy the most elementary book on this subject and you will see electron microscope photographs of clumps of cells differentiating into their roles in life: little arms and legs, fingers and toes.

Look closer at the cells themselves and you will see that each cell is a complete factory. All cellular functions are dependent on the raw materials that are available to fuel them and to provide their building blocks. In babies, the speed at which cells reproduce, grow and repair themselves is phenomenal and all the master control systems that allow this to happen are incredibly finely tuned.

Knowing this will, I hope, engender a deep respect for the process – and the realization that a fundamental difference can be made with nutrition.

❦ SLEEPY HEADS ❦

One of the reasons that babies sleep so much is that they are conserving their energy to channel it into the business of growing.

WHAT IS 'NORMAL'?

This is always a source of anxiety for parents, especially for first-time parents. Firstly, it is necessary to recognize that your child is an individual and what is 'normal' for another child will not necessarily be the same for him. Your health visitor will make regular checks during his infancy and it is important to take advantage of the information that the health visitor makes available.

THE HEALTH VISITOR'S PERSPECTIVE

There is much weighing and measuring in the first few months and there are standard centile charts, provided by your health visitor, that tell you how your child is developing in relation to the average height and weight for his age. The health visitor or nurse will be looking for standard markers including height, weight, alertness, dexterity, coordination, eyesight and hearing acuity. They will also run standard tests for various childhood problems and illnesses. You may find that whilst the Health Visitor's training in paediatric nutrition is helpful for dealing with obvious deficiencies, it is not necessarily geared up to using nutrition as a positive and constructive tool.

💗 WHAT'S IN A CELL? 💗

Each cell has a central 'command' centre called the nucleus, as well as energy production centres called mitochondria. Each has a transportation and storage centre for various cellular products, called endoplasmic reticulum. The protein processing, sorting and delivery systems are called golgi complexes. The cellular waste disposal systems are called lysosomes. All cells are protected by complex phospholipid membranes that are part fat, part protein to keep them waterproof, and yet allow in necessary nutrients via gateways. Depending on the type of cell it is, each has different hormone receptor sites to make it sensitive to specific circulating hormones. If all this were not enough, the cells all produce their own local 'hormones' called prostaglandins. All this activity takes place within each individual cell. Each cell is a miracle in its own right and has an extraordinary set of mechanisms to replicate and to repair itself when damaged.

THE NUTRITIONIST'S PERSPECTIVE

If you are hoping that your children are going to be centre-backs or Amazons, do remember that while nutrition can optimize their potential, there are limits. Genetics play the main part in this story. If both parents are 1.6 m/5 ft 3 in do not be too surprised if your child does not reach much more.

As a nutritionist, I am as interested in symptomatic evidence as developmental markers. What are the child's stools like? Is his skin smooth and plump or dry and flaky? Are there any areas of inflammation or rashes? What are his sleeping patterns? Is the child calm and happy or does he show signs of listlessness or slight hyperactivity? Do his eyes seem bright and clear? Is he able to fight infections well? In other words, what are the markers of good health?

The reason I am interested in these symptoms is that I always come back to my basic precept – if you give the child what he needs to optimum levels, the child's body will have the capacity to operate, at a cellular level, at its peak. Do this and the problem symptoms will not be there. If the symptoms are there, it means that something is not being provided or something is blocking optimum functioning. It also could mean that your child has specific genetic nutritional requirements.

My definition of 'what is normal?' is what is normal for your child, allowing for his individual genetic make-up and giving him the opportunity to develop to his optimum level. There is no other normal – only average; and average is meaningless as far as the individual is concerned.

I say this because averages keep changing. Every 20 years or so, the average height, weight and IQ levels to which our children are expected to conform change – some upward and some downward. All that happens is that a sample of the

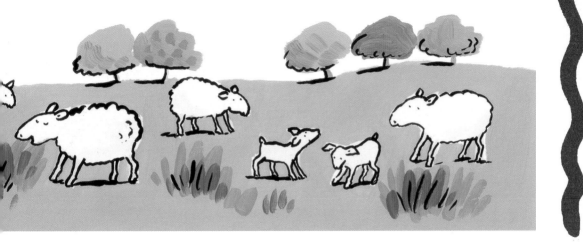

population is taken and statisticians work out what is average at that time. The individual, however, is just that – individual. Determining what is best for the health of your child is a singular task. Averages will be disappointing if your child is 'below par', or they can lead to false expectations if your child surpasses the median figures. Do what is best for your child, and you cannot lose.

There are outward signs that enable you to detect changes in your child's state of health. They could reflect nutritional imbalances, allergies, infections or specific health problems, which may need medical attention – or they could be benign. It is the changes that you need to look for. Some children naturally have pallid skin and others have florid complexions – but if a child moves from one to another for any length of time then it is wise to be alert. The chart (*opposite*) offers some prompts to look for, where a change from one usual condition to another could indicate a need for attention.

There are key dietary factors of which parents need to be aware. Before we discuss these, it is interesting and useful to have an understanding of how your baby's physiology functions. The main systems that I would like to introduce to you on the following pages, and which I feel are the most helpful to know about, are the digestive, nervous and immune systems.

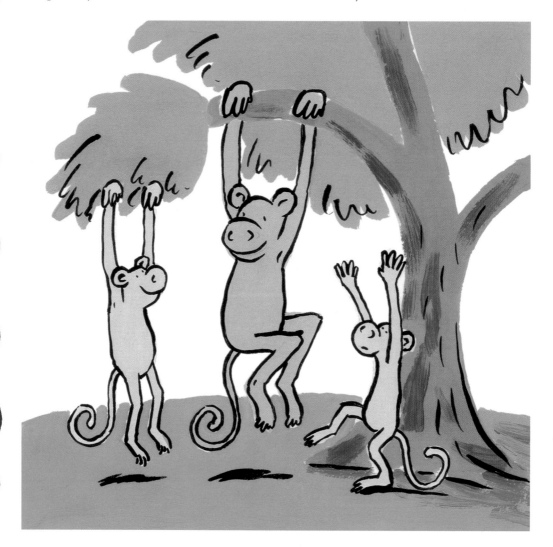

❧ SYMPTOMATIC EVIDENCE ❧
OF INTEREST TO THE NUTRITIONIST

SKIN COLOUR:
Even complexion
Florid
Pallid
Broken veins
Patchy

SKIN TEXTURE:
Smooth and plump
Dry
Cracked
Rashes
Pimples
Areas of inflammation
Bruises easily

EYES:
Normally bright
No circles under the eyes
Circles present when tired
Circles present occasionally
Circles present all the time
Frequent conjunctivitis

APPETITE:
Good
Poor
Excessive
Excessive thirst

DIGESTIVE:
No problems
'Sicky' baby
Excessive wind
Colicky
Frequently bloated abdomen

BOWEL MOVEMENTS:
Bulky and pass easily
Constipated
Loose
Diarrhoea
Lots of undigested particles
Stool colour: mid-brown,
white/yellow, blackish
Mucus in stools
Worms in stools

ENERGY LEVELS:
Energetic
Listless
Boisterous
Overactive
Hyperactive

MOODS:
Content
Passive
Aggressive
Unhappy
Excessive crying
Anxiety
Demanding
Restless

ALERTNESS:
Focuses well
Can be attentive
Interested in surroundings
Disinterested
Listless

SLEEPING PATTERNS:
Regular cycle
Sleeps well
Disturbed nights
Sleeps a lot
Does not sleep much

BREATHING:
Even
Sounds raspy
Mucus in respiratory tract
Difficult to catch breath

IMMUNE SYSTEM:
Fights off infections readily
Takes a long time to fight
    infections
Prone to fevers
Mucus frequently in nose or
    respiratory tract
Prone to allergy symptoms
    (hay fever, eczema, asthma,
    psoriasis)
Comes from family prone
    allergy symptoms
Frequent ear ache

WEIGHT:
Gains weight and height
    steadily
Underweight
Overweight

THE BASIS
OF GOOD HEALTH -
THE DIGESTIVE SYSTEM

A baby's digestive tract is not fully formed and does not reach full maturity until around the age of two years. The mucosal lining of the digestive tract is more permeable than that of an adult and is more porous to proteins in the first year of life. This means that we need to respect the differences between an adult diet and a baby's diet.

The digestive tract is a barrier between the outside world and the body in the same way that the skin is a barrier. Until food is digested and can be absorbed across the digestive wall into the body it is a 'foreign body'. It is only when a molecule is microscopic enough not to do harm that it should be able to cross the barrier. At that point it can be used as a building block or for energy.

DIGESTION

The digestive process actually begins in the mouth where the food is mixed with a carbohydrate-digesting enzyme. The food in the mouth also triggers the release of other digestive enzymes further down the digestive tract. It is fairly pointless talking about the value of chewing food properly when talking about a small child. However, as the child grows up it is worth remembering that chewing food properly is a significant aid to good digestion, and therefore good health.

The stomach in babies and toddlers is very small and can only deal with small portions of food. This is why it is better to feed small children little and often – so a morning and mid-afternoon snack is usually necessary. The stomach is where protein digestion begins to take place, as hydrochloric acid and protein-digesting enzymes are secreted there.

After a while, once it has been sufficiently acidified, the food is released from the stomach into the small intestine. Different types of digestive enzymes, along with bile, are secreted by the pancreas and gall bladder into the small intestine to start the process of carbohydrate and fat digestion. The food then begins to be pushed along the tract and some absorption starts to take place.

The surface of the lining of the small intestine is covered in tiny protrusions called villi and microvilli, which increase the surface area for absorption to allow for maximum uptake of the food eaten. In adults these villi increase the surface area to approximately that of a small football pitch! The villi can be damaged by food allergies, which cause a number of problems – luckily they also repair quite readily if given the chance.

The body's ability to produce a constant supply of digestive enzymes is the most important aspect in ensuring good digestion – after chewing food properly. It is worth noting here that babies do not start to produce one of the most important starch digesting enzymes, amylase, until between four and six months of age, and the enzyme pepsin, which helps to break down proteins, is not produced in the pro rata of adult amounts until the age of about two years. Enzyme production can be helped along by drinking sufficient water and eating a variety of fresh fruit and vegetables (raw or very lightly cooked) to provide the plant enzymes that stimulate our own digestive enzyme production. These valuable plant enzymes are destroyed in the process of cooking foods (*see page 72*).

BACTERIAL BALANCE

The large intestine, or colon, is the end of the process, with some final digestion (by bacteria) and absorption taking place. It is here that most of the water in food is reabsorbed.

In the colon we have billions of resident bacteria, the balance of which is critical to good health. The ideal balance should favour 'beneficial' bacteria which keep the 'bad' bacteria in check. If this balance is disturbed then a number of processes do not take place so well. The bacteria help to digest the last residues of proteins; they help to break down carbohydrate links, failure of which can lead to excess gas; and they produce some vitamins on which we are dependent – particularly B-vitamins and vitamin K. Increased levels of the bad, or putrefactive – the name says it all – bacteria can also be an extra load on the immune system since they produce some toxic byproducts. Good bacteria also maintain the bowels in a slightly acidic state which is necessary to reduce the chances of bowel cancer later in life.

There are around 400 different species of bacteria inhabiting the human bowel. Some of the beneficial bacteria that you may have heard of are acidophillus and bifido bacteria. Babies are born with sterile guts which are colonised by bacteria in the first few days. Breast feeding greatly favours the beneficial bacteria being successfully established.

Good bacterial balance is also supported by eating live 'bio' yoghurt and by a diet with sufficient quantities of fibre, in particular soluble fibre (*see page 49*). Poor bacterial balance can be exacerbated by bottle-feeding, antibiotics, low-fibre diets and excess stress.

Some people worry about giving small children too much fibre, but what is at stake here is the right kind of fibre (*see page 49*). Yes, it will mean more dirty nappies to deal with, but it is never too early to start and lots of dirty nappies are preferable to constipation, irritable bowel, appendicitis, colitis, diverticulitis, or even bowel cancer later in life!

❧ MENTIONING THE UNMENTIONABLE ❧

Stool colour and consistency is not a frequently discussed topic in polite society – until we become parents, and then it is no holds barred on the full details.

There is a wonderful scene in the film *The Last Emperor* (about the Emperor Pu Yi's childhood and life) where the Chief Eunuch examines the baby Emperor's stools in great detail, to determine what his state of health is and what that day's diet should be. I am not suggesting you go to quite this length, but the state of your child's bowel movements will tell you quite a lot about his health and diet. So what is the right colour, consistency and frequency?

Meconium: This is the bowel discharge that all babies excrete in the first day or two. It is a dark-green colour that is not typical of later movements and the first breast milk, colostrum, encourages the excretion of meconium.

Breast-feeding: With breast-feeding, stools will be yellowish and loose. This is completely normal. They should not have a particularly strong smell. You may have to change up to five dirtied nappies a day.

Bottle-feeding: With bottle-feeding stools are darker and more dense than when breast-feeding. They frequently have a stronger smell because of the different bacterial balance in the baby's colon. The reason for this is that bottle-feeding does not encourage the same beneficial bacteria that breast-feeding does.

After weaning: When weaned the colour will vary between light brown and darker brown depending on the food that your child has been eating. The colour should not be whitish or blackish for any length of time – if it is, consult your doctor or health visitor. When you begin to introduce foods with some lumps, rather than fully puréed, you may see all sorts of undigested food in the stools. This is quite normal as it takes time for your child to learn to chew his food properly, and for his digestive enzymes to get up to strength to do the work that his teeth are not doing. The worst offenders are citrus fruit, raisins, unmashed beans, sweetcorn kernels, and whole grains.

The digestive tract squeezes its contents forward by a method called peristalsis. It is designed to do this in the bowels when the stomach fills up with a meal. The implication of this is that your child is most likely to have a bowel movement just after a meal. The ideal number of motions is around two or three a day. This will only happen if your child is getting sufficient fibre in his diet. Most would consider one a day sufficient but twice is daily is better for babies. The reason for this is that the bowels are designed to be extremely efficient at reabsorbing water but, unfortunately, the longer that waste products remain in there, the better the chance for toxic residue to be reabsorbed.

For information on what to do when your child has diarrhoea or is constipated (*see page 124*).

YOUR CHILD'S
AMAZING BRAIN

Even the most relaxed parents harbour secret longings for their offspring to fulfil their mental and creative potential. Although we may try not to, we do spend a lot of time comparing junior's performance with the children of our friends – when did they roll over, first grasp a toy, recognize a face? Watching your child develop is the richest of experiences.

Your child's brain comes equipped with a staggering hundred billion brain cells! All these brain cells reach their full potential when they lay down connecting pathways – a process called arborization; the majority of these vital connections are made after birth. Each nerve is capable of sprouting up to 20,000 branches – it is this that makes the human brain the remarkable complex and integrated web, unique among all the creatures of the planet, that it is. The first two years of a child's life are crucial in terms of creating that potential.

In addition to giving your child every opportunity and a loving environment to help him develop his mental faculties, you have another powerful tool to help develop his brain power to its maximum – the food he eats.

Your child's hundred billion active brain cells enable him to hear, see, taste, smell, feel, touch, talk, walk, think and write. These are complex tasks and the cells need plenty of nourishment to work efficiently and speed messages around the brain and the body. To do this they are surrounded by up to a further nine hundred billion other cells that nourish and sustain the brain. The brain – only 1 kg/2 lb of delicate software – uses a massive 30% of the total available energy.

THINK ZINC
Zinc is one of the most essential nutrients for mental health and is needed to help build those neurone links. In fact it is critical for any anabolic, or growing, process – and guess what your child is doing at such a fast and furious rate from birth onward? Foods rich in zinc include sardines, chicken, small quantities of red meat, cauliflower, asparagus, oats, figs, raisins, brown rice, buckwheat, beans, nuts and seeds.

POPEYE WAS (ALMOST) RIGHT
Iron is very important for the increase in size of brain cells at this early stage. However, while spinach is a reasonable source of iron, it is not very absorbable. More absorbable sources include a small amount of red meat, eggs, brown rice, mushrooms, broccoli, kale and green peas.

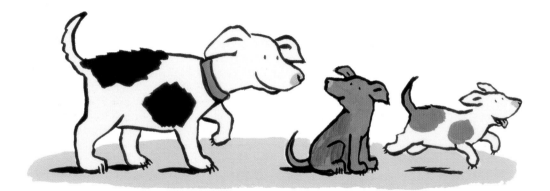

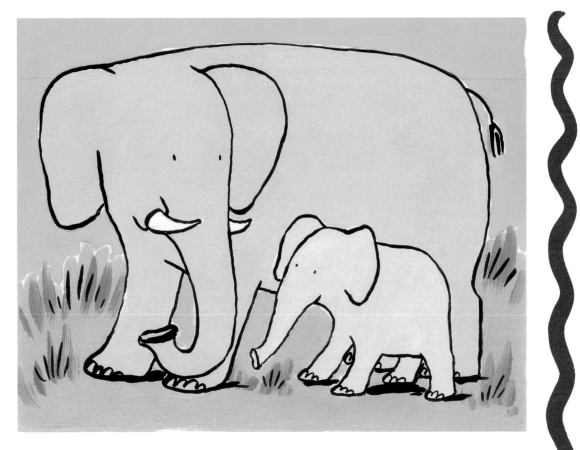

PLENTY OF FISH OILS

Oily fish provide a rich source of 'essential' fats which are intimately involved in building brain potential.

The brain is actually 60% fat, and the types of fats in your child's diet directly affects the availability of building blocks for the brain. Oily fish include mackerel, salmon, sardines, tuna, pilchards and shark among others. Research has consistently shown that the Japanese are, on average, 6 IQ points brighter than their American counterparts – until they emigrate to the USA and stop eating oily fish in favour of the 'Standard American Diet' (SAD!).

A DIET HIGH IN POTASSIUM

Fruit are high in potassium, needed for optimal brain functioning. Half a banana a day will provide all the potassium your baby needs. Other rich sources are potatoes, dried fruit, rye, lentils, peas, molasses and watermelon.

KEEP POLLUTANTS AT BAY

You will also need to take action against some of the pollutants in our environment. Lead is particularly worrying as it is a 'neurotoxin', literally poisoning the nervous system and one in ten children are affected. Luckily, if you follow the advice about zinc you are already reducing the absorption of lead since the two oppose each other (*see page 95*). In addition to the heavy metals (lead, cadmium from cigarettes, excess copper and mercury) many chemicals, of which there are about 60,000 in our environment and 3000 of which are food additives, have an effect on the nervous system. The best advice is to avoid them wherever reasonable and practical. Think seriously about buying organic food if possible and reducing household chemical use. A diet rich in vitamin C (fresh fruit), calcium (ground seeds) and pectin (apples) will help to detoxify – an apple a day really does help to keep the doctor away (*see page 76*).

THE IMMUNE
SYSTEM

The immune system can be thought of as the army that defends your child from a variety of invaders. These include viruses, bacteria, yeasts, foreign proteins such as undigested food molecules, parasites, environmental chemicals and free radicals – highly reactive chemicals and molecules that damage cells.

This army is perpetually patrolling, identifying foreign bodies, marking them, calling in reserves to attack them and then cleaning up the debris after the battle has been won. Signs that the immune system is working well are the ability to produce a fever – viruses die at high temperatures, short-term inflammation at the site of a wound, and short-term mucus production to protect membranes and get rid of waste products. Other signs may be short-term diarrhoea or vomiting to eliminate any undesirable bacteria.

BALANCE
I have used the words 'short term' several times, which is the key to understanding the difference between a balanced situation and one that is out of control and needing attention. A baby's temperature can be highly volatile, but if a fever goes too high, for too long, there is a cause for concern; if inflammation or rashes go on for too long they need addressing; if diarrhoea continues for too long it is dangerous and can lead to dehydration quite quickly; if wheezing is not due to an upper-respiratory tract infection but to asthma, then a resolution must be found. The section on page 122 deals with solutions to some of these problems. The message here is one of awareness – be your child's physician by becoming aware of what is normal and what is spiralling out of control.

Children do seem to have constantly runny noses and upper-respiratory tract infections and it is a relief to know that this is an important part of the process of building up their immunity. Babies are born almost as a clean slate. They have to build up their immunity the hard way by catching colds and diseases and being exposed to bacteria. Their first opportunity to build up immunity is during breast-feeding, which allows them to absorb a large number of antibodies from their mother. Breast-feeding also provides a dose of 'good' bacteria for their digestive tracts.

When children start going to school they catch, on average, a common cold once a fortnight. More than 95 different rhino-viruses are responsible for around 40% of types of colds, and there are many other types of viruses responsible for the rest. By the time the child is an adult he should be much less susceptible as he will have established a measure of immunity to all these types of viruses – cold comfort (forgive the pun) when you are nursing him through yet another infection.

The section "Immunity for Life" (*see page 116*) gives suggestions to help bolster your child's immune system.

ALLERGIES
Strictly speaking, there are two different kinds of allergies – Type I and Type II. Type I is strictly an immune function allergy and includes food reactions, such as peanut, shellfish or strawberry allergies, and airborne and contact allergies. It can result in symptoms such as asthma, hay fever, urticaria, eczema and, even more dramatically, anaphylactic shock.

Type II allergies, on the other hand, are slow-reacting response allergies, or do not involve the immune system at all (as far as we know at the moment). This is the realm of more insidious food intolerance and sensitivity. Allergies are covered in greater detail on pages 96–99.

VACCINATIONS
The debate about childhood vaccinations is a difficult one and I do not propose to cover it as there are much better sources of information (*see page 187*). All I will do here is urge you to support your child's immune system nutritionally (*see page 116*)

once you have chosen a course of action, and after doing your own research and consulting your doctor.

I do believe that a part of the argument for vaccinations is based on statistics that need to be looked at a little closer. My concern is that statistics deal with averages, and the average population is poorly nourished (*see page 60*). If someone is poorly nourished the immune system will not function to its maximum potential and the person will be more susceptible to the worst possible effects of both the disease itself and the vaccination. If you elect to have your child vaccinated, make sure that his nutrition, and therefore his immune system, is in tip-top shape. Similarly, if you elect not to have your child vaccinated, do exactly the same thing, so that if he does catch the disease itself (and it is probably a good idea that he does, to build immunity early in life) the symptoms are likely to be tolerable.

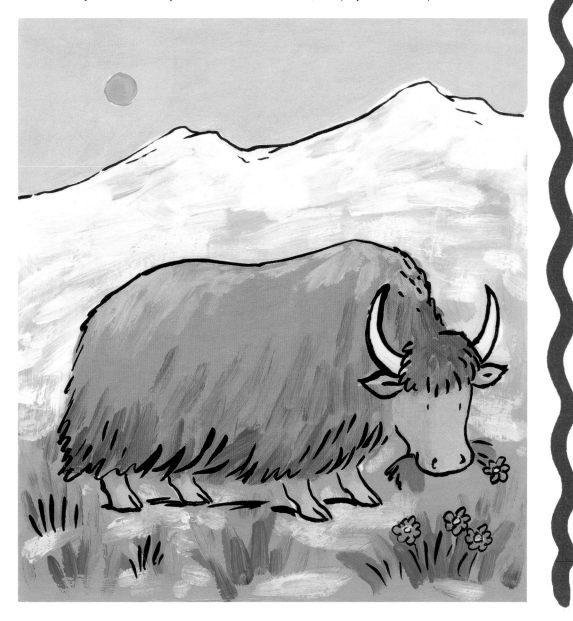

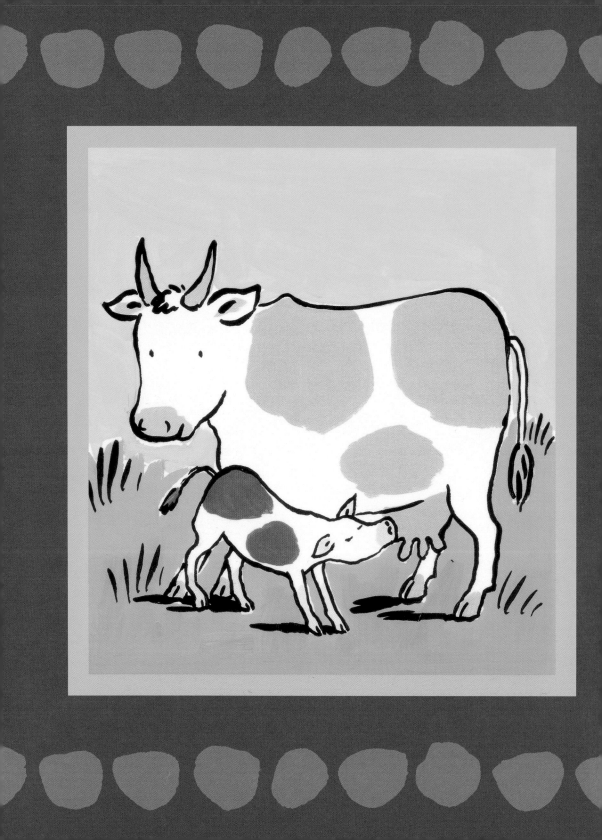

2

THE BREAST & BOTTLE GUIDE

Nature has given us a ready-packaged, perfectly formulated, ready-sterilized, temperature-controlled, easily transportable food for the first part of our children's lives. Why do we think we can do better? I will cover what to do if you elect, or have no choice but, to bottle-feed your child, either exclusively or after a period of time, but as a nutritionist I must come down firmly in favour of breast-feeding. I believe the reasons for not breast-feeding must be very powerful, and not simply ones of convenience or vanity. If this sounds like an extreme statement, then so be it.

BREAST
REALLY IS BEST

Surveys in the 1930s showed that most women breast-fed. By 1975 the level had dropped to only 50% of women. This was a major source of concern and government campaigns were funded to encourage a return to breast-feeding. They have been moderately successful, with an increase now to around 65–75% of babies being breast-fed though often for only 6–12 weeks instead of the recommended six months.

THE ADVANTAGES OF BREAST MILK
There are several things that breast milk delivers that even the best formulated substitute milks do not deliver or are low in.

Colostrum: This is produced in the first three days. It is rich in proteins, minerals and vitamins A, E and B12. These components are not duplicated in formula milks.

Antibodies: Breast milk, especially the early colostrum flow, contains antibodies which coat the gut lining in infants and prevent the absorption of foreign organisms and allergens. These protective substances include secretory IgA, lactoferrin, lysosome and maternal macrophages. These substances are antiallergenic and their effect cannot be duplicated in formula milk.

Digestive lining: It is believed that breast milk helps the baby's digestive lining to mature. Breast milk contains cortisone and epidermal and nerve growth factors, which probably encourage a baby's gut wall to become impervious to foreign proteins faster than bottle-feeding does.

Essential fats: The essential fats vital for the development of the brain, nervous and vascular systems and which help immunity are very low in cow's milk formula and slightly better in Nanny Goat formula milk (a leading brand of infant

formula goat's milk). The first milks to include what are called LCP fatty acids are now available (*see resources*). The importance of these fats cannot be overemphasized. A good indication of the importance of the essential fats to the small infant is that breast-feeding is the only time that we are able to manufacture them and breast milk delivers the ideal balance. Bottle-fed babies are also frequently deficient in DHA (docosahexaenoic acid) and AA (arachidonic acid) fats, both of which are important for nervous system development.

Mineral balance: The mineral balance is different between breast and formula milk. Only breast milk contains the trace elements selenium and chromium. The manganese found in breast milk is 20 times more absorbable than that found in formula milks. Zinc and iron are better absorbed from breast milk due to hormones that are in the breast milk, but which are lacking in formula milk. The calcium in formula milk is less easily absorbed because of the high levels of saturated fats.

Vitamins: Again, the balance is different. Breast milk is rich in the form of vitamin D called 25OHD, which is the best form to avoid rickets (amazingly, in the so-called well-nourished 21st century, rickets is on the increase again). With the exception of Nanny Goat formula, vitamin C is higher in breast milk than in formula feeds.

Enzymes: Only breast milk contains appropriate milk-digesting enzymes.

Bacterial balance: This is radically different with breast-feeding compared to bottle-feeding. Breast-fed babies receive the 'bifidus' factor, which is not available from bottle feeding. The bifidus bacterium helps to protect against other invasive bacteria and establishes healthy gut flora in the baby's intestines.

ESTABLISHING BREAST-FEEDING

Breast-feeding does not always come easily or automatically to all mothers and their babies. Here are a few pointers that could help to increase the success of breast-feeding.

Ideally your baby should be put to the breast as soon as possible after birth. It is at this time that the sucking instinct is at its strongest. The quantity of colostrum produced in the first three days is not all that much and a baby must persevere in suckling through what must seem like lean times. It may be tempting at this time to give a bottle since not much nourishment seems to be coming through, but this early milk is vital for bolstering the baby's immune system and offering a bottle may side-track him from learning to breast-feed.

If your baby is sleeping a lot, do not worry about waking him up to feed. It is important to establish feeding and he will simply go back to sleep again afterwards. To start with, before worrying about a routine, feed on demand to establish suckling as much as possible. If you are eventually going to introduce a bottle or two a day while breast-feeding, do not do this in the first six weeks. This helps to establish breast-feeding as the main source of nourishment. Also a mother's milk flow will be directly related to the amount of suckling taking place, so this initial six weeks is very important for establishing a good flow.

Some parents worry about not knowing how much a baby is getting from breast-feeding. I would advise not worrying as long as your baby is putting on weight – which will be checked by your health visitor anyway.

If you are having trouble establishing feeding do consult your health visitor or a breast-feeding counsellor (*see page 185*).

MIX AND MATCH

If you find that you have to bottle-feed, there are a couple of options to improve the situation. You can, of course, express your own breast milk for use when you are not around. Some people find this easier than others and it does need a certain amount of determination and dedication. Your breast-feeding counsellor will be able to help you if you chose to do this (to find a breast-feeding counsellor *see page 185*).

You can also mix and match. Use some formula when absolutely necessary and breast-feed when, for instance, you return from work. You may need to express some build-up of milk at work when your breasts become full of milk. Eventually this will probably settle down as you adjust to the demand. Initially the let-down reflex has many triggers, including the sight and sound of a baby, but in time it is triggered by suckling alone, as you become more efficient at milk production.

If you have stopped breast-feeding, but decide that formula milk does not suit your child, you may be able to restart as many women continue to lactate for quite a long time after stopping. You will need the cooperation of your child as he may not be willing to do the amount of sucking necessary to get the flow going again, with little early reward for his efforts.

If you do decide to bottle-feed, see *Compensating For What The Bottle Does Not Provide*, page 33, to look at the best way of minimizing the downside.

LOOKING AFTER YOURSELF WHEN BREAST-FEEDING

Breast-feeding has the built-in bonus of helping to return the mother to her pre-pregnancy state. The hormone, prolactin, which is responsible for stimulating milk flow, is also responsible for helping the womb to contract back to its original size. The sheer volume of milk produced (about 600 ml/1 pint a day) also takes a massive amount of energy to produce – this means that if you maintain a healthy diet it is far easier to lose those extra few pounds that the pregnancy may have left you with. Breast-feeding can also provide some family planning benefits as it reduces immediate fertility – however this is not a perfect arrangement and cannot be relied upon.

A major flaw in the argument in favour of breast-feeding is when the quality or quantity of the milk is not good because the mother is not as well nourished as she should ideally be. Research in the USA shows that this is an increasing problem among malnourished educated middle-class mothers. The quality of the breast milk can be so poor from some mothers that their babies fail to thrive. The main problems to look out for are:

❤ If you are suboptimally nourished in nutrients your milk may be lower in some necessary elements. In particular this seems to be the case with essential fats and zinc. Keeping to a low-stimulant, wholefood diet during the pregnancy and during breast-feeding will help to ensure that your milk delivers what it should (*see opposite page for more specific guidelines*).

❤ The milk will provide large quantities of some nutrients to your baby at the expense of your own stockpiles. In particular, in the first eight weeks, huge quantities of zinc are used up as your baby needs it for the massive growth spurt that is happening. Essential fats are also being pumped out in breast milk and it is at this time that mothers often notice that their skin quality reduces or that they get some eczema – all signs of a deficiency in these vital fats.

❤ Milk production uses up a large amount of water, both in the breast milk liquid itself and also in the enzyme process to produce it, and many mothers complain of constipation as they literally dry up. Drinking about 2–3 litres/3½–5 pints of water a day and avoiding dehydrating drinks like coffee, or excess tea or alcohol, usually resolves this.

❤ A major source of concern can come when a breast-fed baby is experiencing a lot of colic or eczema or other disturbances. It is important to rule out food allergies that may be being transmitted in breast milk. The main culprits are usually wheat products, such as bread, cereals, biscuits, pies and pasta, and dairy products (*see page 99*). It is also possible that peanut allergies in children, which can have very bad consequences (*see page 96*) may be linked to the consumption of peanuts by breast-feeding mothers.

❤ It is not fair, in my view, to expect your baby to have a cup of coffee via your breast milk or excess tea or alcohol, so being moderate while breast-feeding is a good idea. I do know one lady who swore that a couple of glasses of wine before a feed put her baby into a deep sleep! While this may seem like a good idea, I would not recommend it because of the effect on the nervous system. Some babies will get windy with too much onion or garlic in the breast milk and very spicy foods will flavour breast milk – I am sure that is why my little boy likes curries so much!

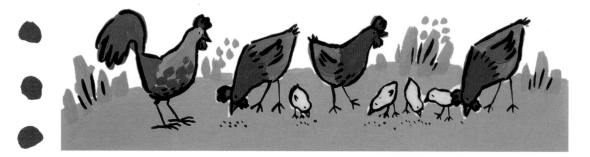

❧ HEALTHY EATING PLAN FOR MOTHERS ❧

I would suggest the following healthy eating plan for most mothers while breast-feeding:

1 Eat plenty of fresh fruit (four pieces a day) and vegetables (two to three portions a day).

2 Eat plenty of fibre-rich foods, such as pulses, beans, lentils, root and green vegetables, and oats. Keep sugars and refined carbohydrates (*see page 48*) to a minimum.

3 Drink at least 2 litres/3½ pints of filtered tap or mineral water a day.

4 Snack on fresh pumpkin and sunflower seeds and fresh nuts like almonds and walnuts for their essential fat and zinc content – chew properly to help digest them.

5 Avoid coffee completely – it is a very strong stimulant. The toxic chemicals in it include caffeine, theobromine and theophylline. Restrict tea to three cups a day, and be very moderate about alcohol intake, say three or four glasses of wine a week.

6 Favour oily fish, white meat and game over formed red meat in your diet.

7 If you suspect your child may be reacting to foods in your diet, avoid them completely for six weeks to see if it makes a difference. Avoid all the main allergens at the same time (*see page 97*). If you avoid the foods one by one, they could be 'masking' each other's allergic signs and you will not discover which ones are causing, or contributing to, the problem.

8 Take a good-quality vitamin and mineral supplement – many brands formulate them especially for lactating mothers. I would suggest that the formulation includes 15 mg of zinc, 10 mg of iron, 500 mg of calcium, 250 mg of magnesium and 1 g of vitamin C. If you do not get enough essential fats from your diet, add a tablespoon of cold-pressed flax oil a day to your food (*see page 77*). As far as price is concerned, you tend to get what you pay for, so buy good-quality brands. I believe that a well-nourished mother will also have less, or no, problems with post-natal blues – at least this has been my experience with the mothers under my care.

9 It may be wise to avoid high amounts of vitamin B6 (in excess of 50 mg per day), and not to be too liberal with the herb sage, as both of these may interfere with breast milk production.

10 Breast-feeding uses up around 500 calories a day, so losing weight is often a bonus for new mothers. However this is not a time to diet, especially as you may find that in so doing you restrict the nutrient quality of your food. See what happens to your weight, and eating healthily will probably mean that your weight will stabilize anyway.

11 One of the most popular misconceptions is that you 'need milk to make milk'. If you are following a dairy-free diet because it suits you or your baby best, there is no chance that your milk flow will be negatively affected.

As I have said, being a milk production factory is an intensive process in terms of energy and this, coupled with interrupted nights, means that you will need to rest. Expect to feel a little tired. If you are eating well and looking after yourself and were reasonably healthy to start with, it will not necessarily be the knock-down-dragged-out sort of tired, but a healthy 'I need to sleep a bit more' kind of tiredness. Listen to your body. I felt so good for the six months after having my little boy, that I know that I took it for granted and overdid it. Keep some energy in reserve and take naps from time to time.

Whatever you do, do not feel guilty about looking after yourself – you deserve it.

THE BEST
BOTTLE OPTIONS

For small children under the age of one year you must always use either breast milk or formula milks which have been modified for human baby consumption. Do not be tempted to use ordinary cow's, soya, goat's or ewe's milk as the milks are not nutritionally complete for small babies and young digestive systems simply cannot handle them. Ordinary cow's milk is too low in iron and vitamin D and too high in the milk protein, casein, for babies. Unmodified cow's milk is good for baby cows but not for baby humans. The metabolism of the excess proteins puts a tremendous stress on the liver and kidneys – the liver has to break down the surplus amino acids and the kidneys have to get rid of the surplus urea created.

If you decide to bottle-feed, there are several formula options available. When making up the formulas, always follow the manufacturers' instructions and do not be tempted to make a stronger or weaker mixture than is recommended. Aim to avoid any milks with added sugar, glucose or corn syrup – your baby does not need these.

INFANT FORMULA COW'S MILK
This is the type of formula milk used by most parents, and there are many brands available at the chemist or supermarket. It has been formulated to be as close as possible to human milk by adding certain nutrients and removing other elements. A part of the protein component, casein, is removed, as is a lot of the calcium, since it is far too dense otherwise for babies. Fatty acids that are found naturally in breast milk are difficult to add to formula milk but the technology is improving and some milks now have LCPs (see resources). A cow's milk that provides some essential fats, and also the only organic milk that I know of, is Babynat, which is imported from France. It does, unfortunately, have maltodextrin (*see page 92*) on its list of ingredients, but if organic is important to you, this is one option. See page 33 for ways to redress the balance between formula and breast milk.

FOLLOW-ON MILK
This is nutritionally a more dense milk for older, or hungrier, babies and provides more calories. The manufacturers also add extra iron, as children need a bit more from around the age of six months. Follow-on milk is more difficult to digest and must not be given to babies before this age.

SOYA MILK
Soya milk seems to be the preferred option for most paediatricians when suggesting that a child goes on a dairy-free diet. It is fairly high on the list of foods that can cause allergies (*see page 97*), so excess use may not be a good idea. The first ingredient listed on soya milk packaging is glucose syrup solids, which is sugar and can set up tooth decay in small developing teeth. Some soya milks have a greater chance of being contaminated with aluminium. Soya milk is high in plant-based phyto-oestrogens. While they are considered to be protective against damaging environmental xeno-oestrogens (from pollution) there is some concern that babies raised on soya milk will be getting many times the quantity of phyto-oestrogens than is advisable.

GOAT'S MILK
Formula goat's milk is better tolerated than most formula milks and the strong 'goaty' taste is eliminated during processing, making it acceptable to young palates. Goat's milk is more digestible than cow's milk, since it coagulates into smaller lumps in the stomach, which are easier for the digestive system to handle. Goat's milk can often be tolerated by infants with a sensitivity to cow's milk, as the gamma-casein that is in cow's milk is absent in goat's milk.

The leading brand of infant formula goat's milk is called Nanny Goat Milk (*see page 185*) and is available from most good health food shops. Nanny Goat formula also has added vegetable oils, which give a better fat profile than cow's milk, when compared to human milk.

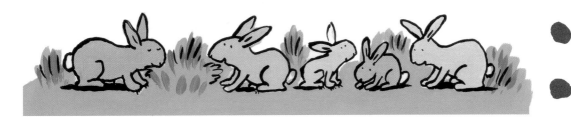

HYPOALLERGENIC FORMULA MILK

If your child proves to be severely intolerant to cow's or soya milk, your doctor can prescribe several types of hypoallergenic formula milks. These are not recommended unless the infant has exceptional problems, which might include severe diarrhoea as a reaction to other milks, failure to thrive or cystic fibrosis.

ROTATING

I have always worked on the basis that, in the same way that it is advisable to have a wide variety of foods in the diet (*see page 61*), it is also a good idea, if not breast-feeding, to alternate between a variety of types of milk. The reason for this is that if your baby is prone to allergies, you reduce the opportunity for them to develop, and at the same time you get the best of all the nutritional options available from the various milks, while minimizing the risk of the downside. As all formula milks have to conform to certain standards of nutrition, this makes rotating them a safe option and they are all suitable from birth. I would suggest rotating the different milks on consecutive days, so one day on goat's milk, one day on soya milk, and one day on cow's milk.

What is not safe is to use anything other than specially prepared infant formulas before the age of one year. Beyond that age you may want to stick to formula milks or begin to add some of the other dairy alternatives in moderation, such as calcium enriched rice milk, oat milk or soya milk, goat's milk or even cow's milk (although I do not recommend it in any quantity – *see page 66*). Whatever you decide to do, I believe rotating the milks is the best option.

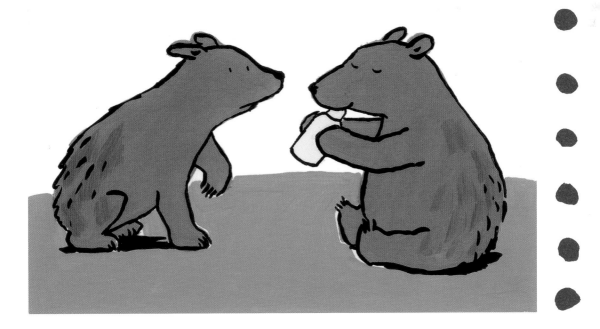

REASONS
FOR BOTTLE-FEEDING

Some parents truly have no choice but to bottle-feed. I would urge those that do have the luxury of choice not to give in to bottle-feeding too readily. A significant number of mothers stop at twelve weeks, but carrying on for six months minimum is best. Reasons why parents might decide to bottle-feed include the following:

Adoption: Obviously in this instance there really is no option but to bottle-feed. Do not worry that you cannot give your child the best start nutritionally, you will be able to help compensate by following the guidelines on the opposite page. And of course, you are giving your new baby the best possible start in every other respect – nothing is as important as the love that you can give your child.

Poor milk flow: This is less likely to happen with a well-nourished mother on a good wholefood diet with a low level of stimulants. (See 'Looking After Yourself When Breast-Feeding', page 28.)

Sore or cracked nipples: This is a common problem and, if you are suffering from very sore, cracked and dry nipples, it will probably take a monumental amount of resolve to persevere with breast-feeding. The first thing to ensure is that your baby is latched on properly. You may think that this comes easily and naturally, but it is probably one of the key reasons why people do not succeed with breast-feeding. If you need more guidance contact your health visitor or one of the breast-feeding organizations listed on page 185. You should also allow the nipples to heal, by only feeding your baby from one breast for a few days or by using nipple shields. As the nipples toughen up the problem usually goes away, but not before a certain amount of discomfort on the part of the mother.

Going back to work: This is probably the most difficult situation to rationalize completely – life is very busy for a working mother at the best of times.

See page 27 for advice on mixing and matching.

Drug treatment: Should the mother have to take drugs of any sort, the doctor may advise against breast-feeding as the drugs will be delivered to the baby in the breast milk. On balance this may be the best advice. If the mother is simply taking a short course of antibiotics, which is quite common if she is experiencing mastitis, then it is probably fine to carry on breast-feeding while making sure that her baby has a course of bifido infantis bacteria to rebalance his bowel flora (see page 122).

Social embarrassment: Yes, even in these enlightened times! You can do a lot to remain discreet and it is worth considering using expressed milk or formula milk in public, while breast-feeding at home in privacy.

Convenience: It is viewed by some as being more convenient to be able to pull out a bottle than a breast. Personally, I cannot think of anything more convenient than breast-feeding.

Self-image: A wry quote I once heard was "I have given my children my womb, I am not going to give them my breasts as well!" You can no doubt guess my thoughts on this comment. Incidentally, if you breast-feed lying on your side on a bed, not only is it more relaxing for most mothers and their babies, but it also creates less of a 'drag' on the breast tissues, helping to keep a better shape. There is also a new problem emerging these days for women who have had cosmetic breast surgery at a younger age, as they are often not able to breast-feed.

Baby blues: If you find breast-feeding so distasteful that you think it will jeopardize your relationship with your child, for instance you may be affected by post-natal depression, then you must follow your own instincts.

❧ COMPENSATING FOR ❧
WHAT THE BOTTLE DOES NOT PROVIDE

I have obviously made a huge noise about breast-feeding, at the risk of alienating parents who have already decided that bottle-feeding is the only option for them. I think that it is important to make a stand about some things and this is one of them. Having taken such a strong line, I would like to say that I also considered bottle-feeding simply because I had had radiotherapy to one breast, due to breast cancer earlier in my life, and was unsure whether I would have sufficient milk from only one breast. This was an unfounded worry, as I might have guessed, since mothers with twins have only one breast per baby and usually have enough milk.

There will be some of you for whom there is no option but to bottle-feed, as already discussed, and for you I offer some suggestions to ensure that your child is optimally nourished. The list of recommendations is quite extensive and may seem a little daunting. If you do not feel you can follow these recommendations to the letter – just do what you can. It is not always possible to measure out drops and powders in the small hours while junior is yelling for a feed.

All of these suggestions are appropriate from birth.

1 Once a day provide the essential fats that the bottle milk does not. Once the milk is ready to give to your baby, add one teaspoonful of cold-pressed flax oil (*see page 77*). Even better than flax oil are the specially formulated oil blends that are designed to have the ideal balance of fats for humans – the brands are called Udo's Choice (after Udo Erasmus, an authority on dietary fats) and Perfect Balance by Higher Nature (*see page 186*). You can also pierce an evening primrose oil capsule and rub it into the soft skin on the inside of your baby's arms and thighs – it is well absorbed across the skin and particularly useful for babies with skin complaints. Older babies can have a Effalex capsule pierced and added to their food.

2 You can buy milk-digesting enzymes (*see addresses on page 186*), which will help with the process of breaking down cow's or goat's milk sugars. Add a couple of drops of these liquid lactase enzymes to the milk when cool and leave them to do their work for a few hours. This should be done with every bottle. There is no point in adding enzymes to soya milk since it does not have lactose (milk sugars) as a component.

3 Keep some powdered infant formula pro-biotics ('good' bacteria), available from Biocare, in your fridge and add half a teaspoonful to the milk when cool, once a day. This helps to rectify the balance of bowel bacteria that is thrown out by bottle feeding.

4 After six months, add a drop of liquid trace minerals, also available from Biocare, to the formula. This provides the selenium and chromium that is lacking in formula milk.

5 Once a day, add 10 mg of vitamin C powder (magnesium ascorbate powder available from Biocare) to the milk when cool. This compensates for the lower level of vitamin C in formula milk compared to breast milk. High levels of vitamin C can cause a loosening of the bowels, but this level should not have any effect. If your baby does suffer some diarrhoea, cut back on the dosage.

6 Bottle-fed babies need more water then breast-fed babies. I suggest offering cooled, boiled water twice a day 10 weeks after birth.

With all of this advice remember that a little is good, but a lot may be not so good – so do not be tempted to double or triple the quantities.

The one advantage that bottle-feeding offers is the opportunity for the father to get really involved. Try to encourage the closeness that is typical of breast-feeding, with lots of body contact and cuddles – from both parents.

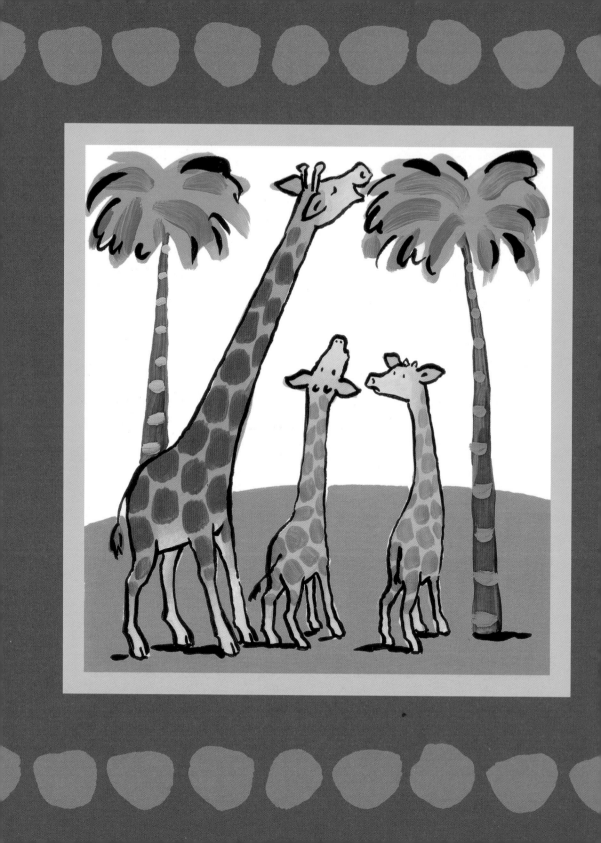

3

WORRY-FREE WEANING

~~~~~~~~~~

Many parents are keen to start weaning their babies as soon as possible, expressing pride at their infant's early progress. However, a baby simply cannot digest anything other than mother's milk or formula before the age of three months – and even that is on the early side. At six months solids need to be introduced as the baby will begin to need more calories than milk alone can provide. So there you have it – between three and six months, although I believe that nearer to six months is ideal. One way or another, your baby will soon let you know if and when he is hungry. If he is dissatisfied with his feed, or chewing at everything in sight then maybe you need to take the hint.

FIRST FOODS
GETTING IT RIGHT

Eating is a new sensation and at first your baby may do no more than just taste the food. Soon he will get the hang of this new activity without too much prompting. Be patient, more may end up on the bib than in his mouth at first. Each new taste needs to be explored. If your baby does not like some tastes, simply try them again a few weeks later. Do not be surprised, too, if something he loves for several weeks suddenly goes out of favour – just try it again at a later date. Tastes change; use single foods first and, as time progresses, you can begin combining to provide a more interesting variety. Early foods must be puréed or finely mashed with no lumps.

The first four months of building up the foods might look like this (*See also page 98 for a detailed list*):

Vegetables: Initially concentrate on the vegetables. In particular, sweet vegetables are usually well received. I would suggest that at this stage you avoid what are called the 'deadly nightshade vegetables' – these are a related family of vegetables, which include potatoes, tomatoes, peppers and aubergines. As the name implies they have compounds to which a young child can be sensitive. On a more positive note, you might like to try any of the following: carrots, parsnips, spinach, sweet potatoes, broccoli, mushrooms, Brussels sprouts, pumpkin, leeks, butternut squashes or swede.

Fruit: The cornucopia is too large to list all fruit individually. They are easy to introduce to babies as they love the naturally sweet flavours. They also mix well with vegetables to give a sweet/savoury variety. Use any fruit that are easy to purée or mash, avoiding any with seeds at this stage, such as pomegranates, kiwi fruit or raspberries. Some parents prefer to give vegetables before fruit in case their child refuses all but the luscious fruit. I do not think it matters hugely, just see what your baby likes. Some people may be concerned that fruit ferment in the stomach while other foods are being digested, and may wish to keep them for separate meals. While this could be a problem for some adults, I am not convinced that it is a problem for the majority of children. In any event this creates a bit of a logistical nightmare. If, however, your child develops wind you can experiment with keeping fruit away from other foods. Many types of fruit can be given raw after 4–5 months, ripe pears and papaya are ideal, and do not have to be cooked as vegetables do, making them an ideal source of nutrition. For the very young, fruit should be peeled, before pulverizing or cutting into fingers to chew on, to minimize the risk of choking on the skin.

Pulses and beans: These can be added at around five or six months and begin to give a little bulk to satisfy a hungry baby. Pulses and beans must be well cooked and blended properly or they can be a little indigestible; for this reason it is best to use canned beans but be sure to choose a no-salt, no-sugar brand, and organic is even better. Lentils are simple to cook but red lentils are the most easily disgestible for babies. All of them – lentils, chickpeas, white beans, flageolets, and so on – combine well with either savoury or sweet ingredients to provide endless interesting dishes.

Rice, quinoa and millet: Baby rice is a staple of the shop-bought baby foods; be sure to use a brand that is organic and free of fillers, such as Organix. However, I would prefer, ideally, to use home-made brown rice, millet, or quinoa (*see Recipe Index*) as they have very low allergenic potential and are a good source of proteins, starches, minerals and vitamins. Grains and cereals other than these should be left until later as they have a higher allergenic potential – these include barley, corn, rye, oats and wheat.

Poultry, meat and fish: These should be introduced in small quantities, preferably keeping red meat to a minimum and concentrating on fish, especially oily fish, poultry and game.

HOW MUCH?

In the first week or so your baby will be able to handle only a teaspoonful or two of mushed-up food at a sitting. You may find that initially he finds it easier to suck some food from your (clean) finger. In time you may learn to think in numbers of ice cubes, as you prepare and freeze food in ice-cube trays (*see page 40*). Your child will increase the quantity slowly – let him decide. Be patient; meal times should not be rushed and your baby will decide when he is full. Maybe he just wants another taste sensation, in which case try a second course – for example a fruit dish after a vegetable dish.

ESTABLISHING SOLIDS

Initially, the food you give your baby will be pulverized to a mushy consistency. He will not be able to deal with any lumps and indeed, for safety against the hazard of choking, you need to be sure that it is completely smooth. Around the age of five to six months babies like to exercise their jaws on everything around, but their food should still be a purée. You can give him some carrot, cucumber or apple sticks to chew on to toughen up his gums, although from the point of view of the risk of choking you may prefer to use teething rings. Teeth usually begin to appear at around six months, and at this time you can pulverize food to a slightly lumpier consistency. Food that encourages chewing helps to develop jaw development and may help to avoid crowded teeth later in life. Never leave babies alone with any food in case of choking.

WHEN TO GIVE UP BREAST OR FORMULA MILK

Ideally, it is desirable to carry on breast-feeding until the age of one, or even later. Certainly, you should keep up either breast or formula milk until

❤ WEANING TO AVOID ALLERGIES ❤

It is all too easy for allergies, or food sensitivities, to be established in a young child. There are three golden rules for reducing the chance of your child developing an allergy, as follows:

1. Follow the sequence of food introduction on page 98 to minimize the risk.

2. Introduce one food at a time and try to keep a food diary, noting down any unusual reactions. If you think your child reacts, avoid the food for a week or two and then reintroduce it to see if the reaction is repeated. It is important to be organized about this; otherwise, if you introduce too many foods at the same time, the results become meaningless and confused. If you notice that any foods provoke a severe allergic reaction, such as difficulty in breathing, swelling of the lips and face, or any other signs of which you are unsure, it is vital that you contact your doctor immediately.

3. Rotate foods as far as possible from day to day. Many allergies are established because of the frequency of consumption. You may feed your child a food for several months and suddenly notice that he starts to have some symptoms like digestive or skin complaints. The best way to avoid this is to rotate foods. For example, do not have the same cereal for breakfast every day: one day have porridge, the next a rice-based cereal, one day a corn-based cereal, and on another day a cooked breakfast.

that age. If I had it my way, from a nutritional standpoint, we would probably carry on breast-feeding until nearer the age of two, but I realize that this is not a realistic option for many mothers. I believe it is around this time that nature intended us to wean our children, as the child's ability to digest milk often begins to decrease.

You may find that your child decides for himself when to give up breast-feeding. This is often more traumatic for the mother than the child – but when they decide to stop, they just do it. I was determined to carry on breast-feeding until my son was well into his second year, but at 10 months of age – with no formula bottles to tempt him – he just decided to stop and gave me gentle warning bites every time I tried to persuade him otherwise. So much for theory!

The conventional wisdom is that small children do not thrive best on solid food alone, and need some milk up to the age of two. Government guidelines state that it is safe to introduce ordinary cow's milk into the diet at the age of one year. I would prefer to see a wider range of nutrients coming from a variety of foods, and for milk to take a second place in the diet after the age of one, and then preferably from breast or formula milks rather than cow's milk. To repeat myself, you are raising a human infant and not a calf. See Chapter 2 for more information on breast milk and formula milk.

WHEN HE STARTS TO FEED HIMSELF

This is where all hope of control can go out of the window. Luckily, around the age when your child begins to be interested in feeding himself, his need for calories takes a bit of a dip. I say 'luckily' because a lot of food will end up on the floor! You will probably have to allow more time for meals than you have so far, and be prepared for him to be more pernickety as he has the option of whether to put something on the spoon or not. Trying times indeed! Part of the trick is to stay relaxed and keep distractions to a minimum.

💚 IS IT HUNGER AT 2 A.M.? 💚

The greatest bane for just about every new parent that I have ever spoken to is interrupted nights. Some common reasons for a baby waking and crying are thirst, dirty nappies (wet nappies get very cold at night), being too cold or too hot, not feeling well, lack of an established pattern or sleeping too much in the daytime. Another possibility to consider is hunger, especially if he has a pattern of waking every night at the same time. A few things to try might be:

1. Wake him up for a breast-or bottle-feed before you go to bed. This may seem cruel when your child is so dozy, but it is a lot less cruel than you getting no sleep – simply because your child gets to catch up during the following day and you probably don't.

2. Try one of the 'soporific' foods as a late snack – porridge, brown rice, chicken and turkey are all great for this.

3. If you are following the advice in this book and not giving your child foods that induce poor blood sugar handling (*see page 63*), you should have a reduced risk of him waking because of a blood sugar dip at 2 a.m. in the morning.

COOKING
FOR BABIES - SAFETY FIRST

For at least the first six months of your baby's life it is important to sterilize all bottles and feeding equipment. You can buy special steam sterilizing equipment, but perfectly good alternatives are either to boil feeding equipment in a large pan for 10 minutes, or to put it into the dishwasher on a normal cycle. Boil the teats separately in a covered pan, making sure there are no air bubbles trapped in the nipples.

Babies are more vulnerable to food poisoning than adults and so care must be taken to avoid bacterial growth on foods:

❤ Leftovers should be frozen for the maximum safe time at below 0°C/32°F (*see page 40*). Frozen foods should be thoroughly defrosted before cooking and you should not refreeze food.

❤ If using commercially prepared baby foods only the amount that is likely to be used in one meal should be transferred to a feeding dish using a sterilized spoon. The remainder can be refrigerated in the jar, properly sealed, for the following meal. Do not keep it for longer than the next meal.

❤ Small children are more susceptible to the really nasty problems presented by listeria and salmonella. For this reason do not give a young child soft, unpasteurized cheeses or soft egg yolks.

❤ Never cut any food (bread, fruit, vegetables) on a board that has had uncooked meat on it previously. Scrub wooden chopping boards really well after use and let them air dry properly. It is even better to use rigid plastic chopping boards which do not promote bacterial growth.

❤ Cook fish and meat thoroughly to kill off any possible parasites.

❤ Wash fruit well and, if not organic, peel fruit for small children. It is a shame to do so as the best nutrients are just under the skin, but it is the safest course. Recent government guidelines give this advice, as there can be a build-up of farming chemicals that can cause stomach cramps in small children. Another reason to peel fruit is that very young children can choke on fruit skins.

❤ Always wash hands before handling and making up bottles or handling food. Ensure the whole family, and anyone caring for your children, has it instilled in them to wash their hands with soap – water alone will not do – after going to the toilet or changing nappies.

THE BASIC EQUIPMENT
There is a bewildering array of equipment available to cook for your newborn baby. All manner of sterilizing units and grinders will stare out at you from shop shelves. However you can usually manage perfectly well with what you probably already have in your kitchen. What is listed here is the basic minimum that you need, along with a few useful extras.

Blender, liquidizer, food mill or sieve:
You probably have at least one of these already. If not, an inexpensive food mill will be more than sufficient as you need to purée food for your baby's first few months only. After that you will be mashing and chopping the food. I particularly like a tiny baby food processor, which was quite inexpensive and after being used for baby food had a follow-on life chopping small quantities of herbs, nuts and seeds.

Steamer, colander or sieve with pan and lid:
I use my steamer all the time; however, a sieve over a pan filled with a little water, with the pan lid on top of the sieve to stop the steam escaping, does just as well. You can also purchase multi-level steamers which allow you to cook several foods at a time.

Grater: Using a grater is a good way to serve root vegetables or as an alternative to finely chopping foods for toddlers.

Small pan: This is useful for heating up small quantities of food.

WEANING CUPS, SMALL CUTLERY AND UNBREAKABLE PLATES

Weaning cups that close properly are widely available and are a great relief to any parent whose child decides to use the cup as a watering can. Cutlery designed for small hands is much easier to use and great fun for a toddler. My little boy thoroughly enjoys pouring his own drink from a play teapot into a tea set. It is fun and instils a sense of responsibility about not tipping his drink all over the table.

STORAGE METHODS

Nowadays we are used to convenience foods being readily available and yet, with just a little forethought and planning, healthy eating need

not preclude such convenience.

Freezing: Freezing is a great standby for parents. It conserves most nutrients and is an excellent storage method. When your baby is small it is helpful to have lots of ice-cube trays to freeze small portions of food. The cubes can be turned out into storage boxes to free the ice-cube trays for the next batch. You can cook especially for the freezer, or freeze leftovers. Make sure to label and date the boxes accurately, as everything looks the same when frozen. Do not freeze made-up baby's formula, although you can freeze small quantities of expressed breast milk in special sterile plastic containers, for a maximum of six months.

Dried foods: These are a good resource and nutritionally sound, but make sure they do not go stale. Cereals are especially vulnerable as they will often get microscopic bugs in them if they are stored for too long. I suggest that you store them in airtight containers labelled with 'use by' dates. Dried beans, grains, pulses, pastas and crackers are all good to keep in your larder.

Canned foods: These are always tempting but are really a compromise standby. There are good and bad canned foods, and knowing the difference is a good idea (*see opposite*). The majority of canned foods are processed to the point that there is no nutritional value left at all and, as a general rule, I would suggest avoiding them. Additionally, the cans themselves can leach undesirable chemicals into the food. The problem of tin solder has been resolved, but it now appears the plastic coatings that line the cans are leaching oestrogen-like chemicals. One solution is to use foods packed in glass jars, as many baby foods are. Other foods in glass jars are not as common in the UK as they are in some European countries such as France. The final damning point about canning is that sugar and salt are frequently used, and it is a good idea to avoid these.

❦ FREEZING TIMES ❦

The following are maximum suggested freezing times for foods kept at 0°C/32°F:

Beef or lamb, cooked	4 months
Ham or pork, cooked	1 month
Poultry, cooked	3 months
Fish, cooked	2 months
Vegetables, purées	1–2 months
Fruit, purées	1 year
Bean, lentil, pea soups	2 months

❧ USEFUL CANNED FOODS ❧

Some canned foods can be useful standbys, especially the following items:

Canned sardines, tuna, salmon, mackerel and pilchards: Ideally these should be packed in olive oil or tomato. The useful essential fats (omega-3s) are still largely intact (apart from Tuna).

Beans (white, flageolet, pinto etc.), lentils and chickpeas: These still have their mineral and fibre levels. Place the beans in a sieve and rinse well under running water. As they are already well cooked, they are often better tolerated by small children than home-cooked beans and pulses. In fact red kidney beans, which contain toxic lectins, are much safer canned than taking the risk of not cooking them properly. Check for and avoid added salt and sugar.

Baked beans: There cannot be a household with a child that does not have a can of baked beans lurking in the cupboard. Buy the organic reduced sugar and salt variety from your health food shop – more expensive but worth it.

Tomatoes: A useful standby for casseroles, soups and stews (although I use fresh whenever possible as they taste better). Canned tomatoes, without added salt and sugar, will deliver lycopene, an antioxidant.

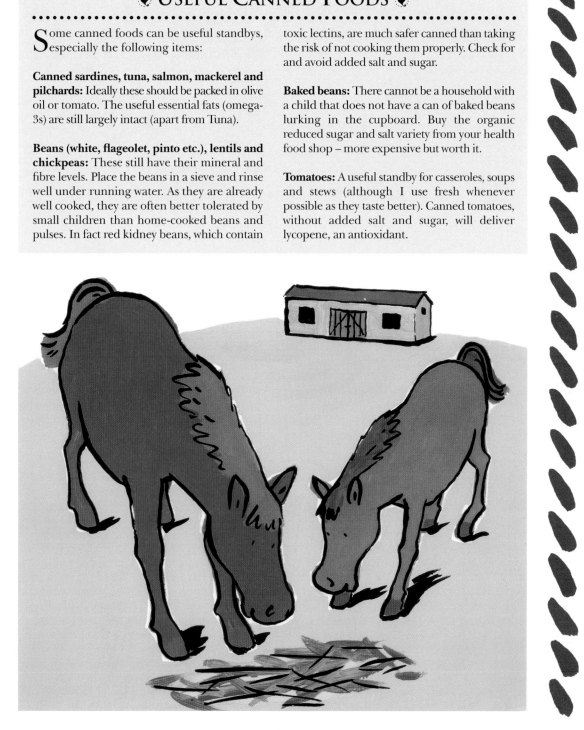

COOKING
METHODS

RAW FOODS

It may seem strange to talk about raw food in a section about cooking, but I have devoted a whole section to this subject (*page 74*) and so this is just a little reminder. Raw fruit and vegetables deliver vitamins, minerals and enzymes so it is a good idea to offer these to your children as often as possible. They also educate your child's palate to enjoy fresh foods. Depending on the food and the age of your child, either mash with a fork or use a mini-grinder. You can also prepare fresh juices (*see page 71*), and older babies can pick up vegetable and fruit sticks.

STEAMING

Steaming preserves the nutrient content of foods better than most other cooking methods and ideally vegetables should be slightly crisp and not soggy. The taste of steamed vegetables is far superior to boiled vegetables. Because it is easier not to overcook when steaming, compared to boiling, more vitamins are preserved and as the vegetable is not soaked in the water fewer minerals are leached out. Fish can also be steamed very well as this method helps to retain the delicate flavours. Be careful not to scald yourself when steaming.

BOILING

I tend to use this method for foods that do not lose many of their nutrients to the water as they have a skin to protect them, for example peas, beans and lentils, sweetcorn, whole butternut squashes and whole potatoes with their skins on.

BAKING

The nice thing about baking is that you can do several dishes at the same time, and stock up the freezer for days when you do not have time to cook. As a cooking method it is quite good as you do not need to use large amounts of fat, compared, for instance, with frying. Baking is particularly good for oily fish as it uses lower temperatures than the hob or grill and so preserves more of the good essential fats. Some vegetables taste particularly good when baked, especially the Mediterranean vegetables that are so colourful: aubergines, courgettes, peppers and red onions. Carrots and other root vegetables will caramelize, making them very appealing to small children. Most people use aluminium baking foil to cover dishes while baking. However, to keep exposure to aluminium to a minimum, I recommend that it is used in such a way that it does not touch the food – create a sort of pocket instead.

GRILLING

When grilling at very high temperatures the food will be denatured, or damaged, quite quickly. I prefer to set the grill on a lower setting and place the grill pan further away from the flame or element so as to cook more gently. Grilling uses less fat than frying and can be good for browning food. However, I do not recommend a lot of 'browned' – or burnt – food for children as the food really is fairly lifeless then, and may be potentially carcinogenic. I would not give a child food from a barbecue too often, for the same reasons.

FRYING

Frying can use a lot of oil and high temperatures. It is better not to fry as a matter of course. Use butter or olive oil, for frying. When you fry with other oils you damage most of what is useful and good about them and create some harmful byproducts.

STIR-FRYING

This is a useful method as it uses only a tiny amount of oil and the vegetables are usually crunchy and not overcooked and I would recommend experimenting with this method if you have never tried it. You can also steam-fry, using a little water instead of oil, or a mixture of olive oil and water in a household plant sprayer. When you have finished the stir-fry add some cold-pressed walnut or sesame oil, to taste, about 1 tablespoonful – as you would a salad dressing. This way you really get to savour

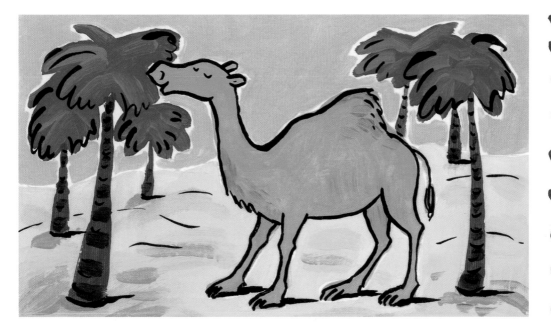

the different tastes, and you get all the nutritional benefit of the oil.

❧ SMOKED AND CURED FOODS ❧

People very rarely do their own smoking, but there are quite a lot of smoked foods on offer so it is worth mentioning. Smoking enhances the flavour of foods quite seductively. It does, however, produce carcinogens and I would avoid giving a child too many smoked foods. Once, or at most twice, a week would be the maximum and then preferably when there are other benefits such as the essential fats in smoked fish. So, for variety and ease, I would give some smoked mackerel or herrings or, if you are feeling rich, smoked salmon (the trimmings are reasonably cheap and just as delicious), but I would generally avoid bacon, ham, sausages and salamis, which are particularly high in the preservative sodium nitrite. Eating a varied diet, rich in fruit and vegetables, should provide damage limitation against the possible negative effects of some smoked foods in the diet.

MICROWAVING

Microwaving is generally considered quite safe, as long as there is no leakage of energy from damaged equipment. For this reason pregnant women are advised to stay away from microwaves.

Microwave ovens work by agitating molecules of animal and plant tissue, which generates heat and cooks the food. Studies show that microwaving preserves the vitamin content of food better than most cooking methods. There is at present very little published research questioning the safety of microwaving from a nutritional standpoint, but I still remain suspicious of any process that oscillates molecules, in view of the delicate balance of the structure of molecules in foods.

In a recent test two groups of volunteers ate exactly the same vegetable-based meal, one lot prepared in a conventional oven and the other lot cooked in a microwave. The results showed that the blood composition of the group eating the microwaved meal was significantly different when compared to the group eating the conventionally prepared food. They had raised cholesterol levels, increased white blood cell counts and lowered haemoglobin values, all of which are findings that should cause some concern.

The jury is still out, and more research needs to be done, but nevertheless I have chosen not to own a microwave.

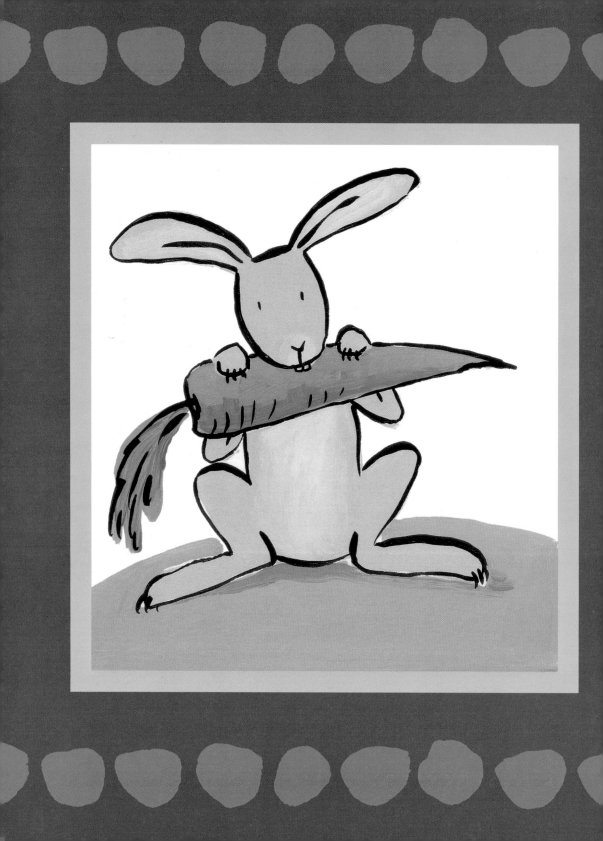

4

NUTRITION BASICS

Here we will look at the main components of food and how they contribute to health. There are around 47 essential nutrients – nutrients that we cannot manufacture, but must get from our diet. These include between eight and eleven amino acids or protein building blocks – the number is dependent on whether we are adults or children – two fats, thirteen vitamins, and twenty to twenty-one minerals.

WHAT DOES
OUR FOOD DELIVER?

Our food, in its natural state, delivers seven principle elements: proteins, fats, carbohydrates, fibre, water, vitamins and minerals. The possible variations of these are many, and the balance and types of the components make the food either useful, useless or damaging. Understanding the difference is the basis of knowing how to make your child's diet work for the best possible result.

PROTEINS

Proteins are made from amino acids and it is these amino acids that are the basic building blocks of all cells – about 17% of our body weight consists of proteins. Not only are all our cells made from proteins, but so are the matrix of our bones, our hormones, our nerve chemicals and enzymes.

Yet the body does not need a huge amount of protein from our diet since we have the fantastic ability to manufacture proteins according to our needs from the 'pool' of amino acids that we have stored in our livers. Dietary guidelines suggest that we need 12–15% of our calorie intake from proteins and yet, at a time when we are growing at the fastest rate – the first six months of life, Mother Nature provides only about 1.5% protein in breast milk.

An adult will turn over about 300 g of protein a day, but does not need more than 40 g a day from food – about the amount you get in two portions of fish or chicken. It is actually very hard to be deficient in protein, on a Western diet, as grains also contribute significant amounts. The problem is much more likely to be one of excess protein. Protein-dense foods include meat, milk, cheese, eggs, pulses, beans, grains, mushrooms, soya, tofu, quinoa, nuts and seeds.

FATS

Fats are used for much more than simply laying down padding, and a baby needs a good amount of the right types of fats. Polyunsaturated fats are used for cell structure, to provide flexibility and protection, for many of our hormones, and for brain development and nerve protection. Sixty per cent of the brain consists of fats – but not just any fats, the type is important. There are three types of dietary fats: saturated, monounsaturated and polyunsaturated fats

Saturated fats

These come mostly from animal products and are solid at room temperature. They include butter, cheese, milk fat, meat fat and eggs. A vegetable source of saturated fat is coconut butter. Polyunsaturated margarines, which have been hydrogenated, become 'dishonourable' members of the saturated fat family. They have been processed from liquid oils to be solid at room temperature, and in so doing have had most of their health benefits destroyed and a few negative effects added for good measure. I do not advise using these margarines. Hydrogenated fats can also be found in any processed food that has used vegetable oils in the manufacturing process. The worst offender are foods such as potato chips, and sweet and savoury pies and pastries.

Saturated fats are used by the body for fat storage as an energy reserve and the body has the ability to make all the saturated fats it needs from carbohydrates. A moderate amount of saturated fat is fine, but again we have a tendency, following a Western diet, to have far too much saturated fat and not enough of the unsaturated variety. Of the saturated fats, butter or coconut butter are the best for cooking with, although it is probably best not to develop a taste for spreading with them or using them to flavour vegetable dishes, as this is where the habit of excess begins.

Too much saturated fat in the diet contributes to most of our killer diseases, as well as the inflammatory diseases like arthritis, later in life. In childhood, if taken to excess, they can be a factor in the development of eczema and asthma – two more inflammatory diseases.

Monounsaturated fats

These comprise a small group that includes olive oil. Because olive oil is almost saturated, but not quite, it is quite stable when heated. It is therefore a good fat to use for cooking as it is not very readily 'denatured' and so remains a healthy option though it should not be heated to smoking point. Olive oil is best bought as cold-pressed, extra-virgin oil – the darker the colour, the better it is for your child. Later in life he will thank you – countries that have a high intake of olive oil have lower risks of all the main age-related diseases. Keep your olive oil in a cool dark place to keep it at its peak – do not leave it standing next to the cooker.

Polyunsaturated fats

These are the main health givers. They can be found in fresh nuts and seeds and their oils, vegetables and oily fish like mackerel, sardines, tuna and salmon. Two of these fats are termed 'essential' fats and are called linoleic and alpha-linolenic acid – also known as omega-6 and omega-3 fats. What is meant by 'essential' is that we cannot manufacture them and must get them from our diet. Required by every cell in the body for normal functioning, they are essential to life and without them we are subject to deficiency diseases. It is these fats that our body uses for vital processes like cell membrane structure, hormones and nervous tissue.

There is much confusion about the best way to get these fats in our diet. For instance, food manufacturers will use the term 'high in polyunsaturated fats' when in fact they may have been processed to the point when they do more harm than good. The best way to make sure you get these fats is to use cold-pressed oils, like sunflower, sesame, safflower or flax oil, or fresh nuts and seeds. It is also important not to cook with them, as heating them destroys most of their health benefits, and in damaging them, creates harmful compounds. (As already stated, for cooking it is best to use olive oil or a little butter. Fresh seeds and nuts become rancid quickly, so it is important to buy in small quantities from suppliers who have a good turnover and who do not let them get stale on their shelves. As with the oils, these are ideally kept refrigerated.

Finally, there are the fish oils. Many long-suffering children of earlier generations were given cod-liver oil – and with good reason. It is the fish oils that we seem to be lacking most of all, and they are very important in babies for brain development. They provide the next stages in the alpha-linolenic, omega-3 series – called EPA (eicosapentanoic acid) and DHA (docosahexanoic acid). I would not advise, nowadays, using cod-liver oil to excess since, for small children, the oil from the flesh of the fish rather than the liver is probably a safer option. Liver oil may have high levels of toxins; also, with high doses, you could overdo your child's vitamins A and D requirements. If you are a vegetarian, flax oil is an alternative source of the omega-3 series fats.

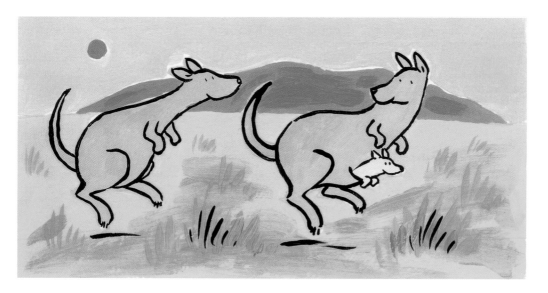

❧ ESSENTIAL FATS ❧

	FEATURES	MAIN FUNCTIONS	FOOD SOURCES
LINOLEIC ACID Derivative GLA (gamma linoleic acid) found in evening primrose oil, borage oil, blackcurrant seed oil, starflower oil	Must be derived from diet; easily destroyed by heat, light and long storage; non-toxic, but excess may show some symptoms	Used in cell walls for protection and flexibility; used for hormone production; makes anti-inflammatory substances (and some inflammatory)	Fresh nuts and seeds; cold-pressed sunflower oil, safflower oil, sesame oil, corn oil, almond oil, grapeseed oil, rice bran
ALPHA-LINOLENIC ACID Derivatives EPA and DHA found in oily fish	Must be derived from diet; easily destroyed by heat, light and long storage; non-toxic	Used in cell walls for protection and flexibility; used in brain structure and for nerve protection; used for hormone production; makes anti-inflammatory and anticoagulatory substances	Cold-pressed flax oil, pumpkin seeds, soya beans, walnuts and their oil. Oily fish such as mackerel, salmon, sardines and tuna.

CARBOHYDRATES

Carbohydrates are our main source of fuel. There are two types: refined and complex.

All carbohydrates finish up as glucose in the blood. The key issue is how quickly they end up as glucose. Too quickly and they have a detrimental effect; nice and slow and energy is available on tap, as needed. The brain uses about 30% of available glucose and since it is such a vital organ, it is given priority over other energy needs. So a nice steady blood glucose level can contribute to nice even moods as the brain is kept nourished optimally. Any harassed parent will understand the benefit of this in a child!

Refined carbohydrates:

Examples of refined carbohydrates are white bread, white rice, peeled potatoes, instant hot cereals, white pasta, most biscuits, most crackers, cakes made with white flour, most pie crusts and sugar.

Refined carbohydrates are a man-made invention and are what is left when the carbohydrate has been stripped of its fibrous elements. During this process many of the nutrients, vitamins and minerals are also stripped out. It is because of this that sugar is described as providing 'empty calories'. In other words these are calories that have no nutritious value at all – no building blocks that the body can use.

Complex carbohydrates:

Typical complex carbohydrates are wholemeal bread, wholegrain cereals, porridge oats, brown rice, jacket potatoes, sweet potatoes in their skins, wholemeal pasta, oat or rye crackers or crackers that specify they are wholewheat and wholemeal pie crusts.

Complex carbohydrates are the form that our bodies can use best. They are a complete package of calories (or energy), vitamins, minerals and fibre. Because our system has developed to use fuel in this form we can metabolize, or burn, the energy at a steady rate. This means that we get an even energy and mood balance, instead of being subject to peaks and troughs. Children in particular benefit from stable energy levels – dishing out refined carbohydrates, and especially sugar, is a bit like giving your child rocket fuel.

FIBRE

Until fairly recently it was considered that fibre was simply the waste product of carbohydrates, and consequently was not needed. It is true that it contributes no nutrients and is eliminated. However, it is of major importance in slowing down the release of sugars into the bloodstream, and in maintaining the health of the digestive tract by, effectively, massaging it and giving it something to work on. A good level of fibre in the diet, especially soluble fibre, is associated with lower risks of cardiovascular disease and diabetes and all the 'Western' digestive disorders such as irritable bowel, diverticulitis, constipation, haemorrhoids, colitis and some cancers.

There are two types of fibre, insoluble and soluble, and we need both. A rich source of insoluble fibre is wheat and wheat bran. However, the habit many people have developed of sprinkling spoonfuls of wheat fibre on to cereals is not the answer, as we also need the soluble fibre. Too much insoluble fibre can be too aggressive as it is an irritant to the walls of the digestive tract. It is particularly not recommended for small children.

Soluble fibre tends to go stringy when cooked, for example oats and fruit. A good amount of soluble fibre is highly beneficial and leads to good, bulky stools – there is a saying I particularly like: 'large stools, small hospitals'. Good sources of fibre include oats, pears, raspberries, figs, prunes, peas, lentils, beans, chickpeas, sweet potatoes, yams, buckwheat and brown rice.

WATER

This is the forgotten nutrient. We are composed of 65% water – even our bones are 25% water. As well as keeping us hydrated at a cellular level, it is

❧ NO GO WITHOUT H₂O ❧

Water is the second most important nourishment for the body. We can go quite a long time without food but we can survive only minutes without air and two or three days without water.

important not to forget that all our enzymes – the billions of chemical reactions that take place daily at every level in the body – are entirely water dependent. If there is not enough to go around, some will not be working optimally.

Call me fussy but I prefer my child's water to be as unpolluted as possible and, as a minimum, would recommend that water is filtered before boiling for an infant. This will remove the majority of the heavy elements and pollutants that may be in your drinking water. Other alternatives are good-quality bottled waters, water distillers or reverse osmosis water purifiers. The only mineral waters to avoid with small children are carbonated waters as they have too much gas for a little digestive tract.

Because, as adults, we are used to drinking a 'drink' we often feel that water is somehow unpalatable – and we may pass that preference on to our children. Yet, in my experience, children who are used to drinking water from early on, will be quite happy to do so and will ask for it by name instead of juices and sodas. Our hunter-gatherer ancestors did not reach for a cola or juice when thirsty or, even worse turn to coffee, they went to the nearest source of clean water. A taste for water is one of the greatest gifts you can give your child. It is truly health giving.

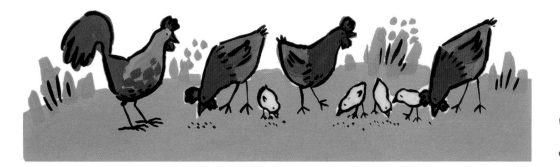

VITAMINS
AND MINERALS

The definition of a vitamin is that it is vital to sustain life and cannot be synthesized by the body – it must be obtained from our diet. Minerals, by definition, also have to be acquired from our diets. The vitamins in our food have been synthesized by the plants or animals that we eat and the minerals have been absorbed by plants from the earth in which they are grown.

Vitamins can be divided into two major groups: fat soluble and water soluble. Fat-soluble vitamins need sufficient fats in the diet to absorb them. They can be stored in the liver and because of this there is the potential to overdose on them. Water-soluble vitamins are generally very safe as they are excreted and not stored. Some vitamins are considered semi-essential as we have the ability to manufacture some of our requirements.

Minerals are classed as either macro-minerals, which are needed by us in large quantities – such as calcium, magnesium and phosphorus for bones, or trace minerals, which are needed only in tiny quantities, for example zinc, selenium and chromium.

If you ask the average person what these substances are for, the answers are normally fairly predictable: calcium for bones, vitamin C for colds and scurvy, carrots (vitamin A) for eyes, vitamin D against rickets. This is largely the way we are taught to think about vitamins and minerals at school – each one helps to counter a major deficiency disease, and such diseases can be avoided by a diet that provides the basic amount of these nutrients. Government agencies set RDAs (Recommended Daily Allowances) and RNIs (Recommended Nutrient Intakes) after establishing what is needed to avoid major deficiency diseases.

MULTIPLE ROLES

This widespread way of viewing nutrient replenishment solely as a means of averting deficiency diseases has a major inherent problem: by taking this approach the more subtle aspects of nutrients contributing to health and well-being are missed. The truth is that all these nutrients have a multitude of roles and they are all completely interdependent. All our body processes work under the influence of enzymes – every breath you take, every thought you have, every beat of your heart, every meal you digest. And all enzymes need vitamins and minerals to work.

Just take one process – the production of energy. I pick this one because most of us do not have enough and all children use huge amounts of it. If you think about it, energy is used for growing, repairing tissue and all body functions. The 'energy cycle' in every cell in the body uses up the following nutrients: Vitamins B1, B2, B3, B5, B6, biotin, folic acid, C, CoQ10, and the minerals iron, magnesium, zinc, manganese and copper.

ANTIOXIDANTS

The antioxidants are worth a special mention as they are so vital. They protect against oxidative damage to tissues, in the same way that lemon juice, which contains vitamin C, will stop a halved apple from going brown (oxidizing) on contact with the air. The main antioxidants are the vitamins A, beta-carotene, C and E and the minerals selenium and zinc. In study after study, these nutrients have been shown to be instrumental in reducing the risk of degenerative diseases, such as cancer and heart disease, in later life. And the time to start stocking up with these protective nutrients is in childhood. They have a major role in supporting the immune system and protecting against asthma. There are also a number of other 'non-essential' antioxidants – meaning that they are not essential nutrients which we must get from our diet. However, there is more and more evidence that they have very important protective roles (see Phyto-nurients page 72). Antioxidants also work synergistically. This means that they all enhance each other's performance – a little of each is far more powerful that a lot of just one of the antioxidant nutrients.

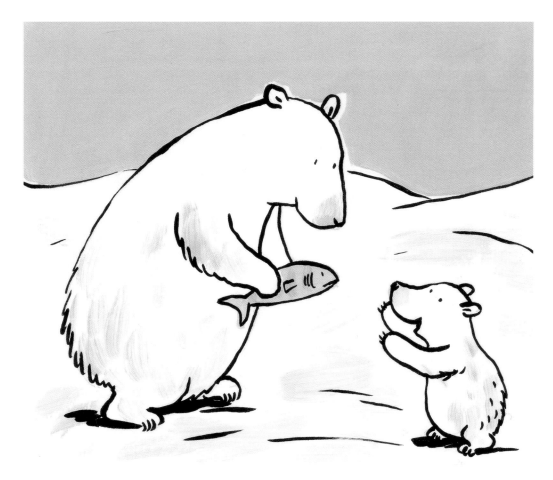

So you can see why getting a good amount of a wide range of nutrients is so vital. The best way to get them is to have a varied diet from as 'pure' a source as possible – organic and unprocessed.

RDAs VERSUS SONAs

The RDAs (Recommended Daily Allowances) have been set by governments to establish levels of nutrient intake that ensure that the general population does not suffer from the deficiency diseases such as scurvy, beriberi and pellagra. You will often see these RDAs quoted on the sides of, for instance, cereal packets which state that the product provides a percentage of the RDA for a given substance. On this basis they have been successful because the general population does not, for the most part, have a problem with deficiency diseases (although they are now slightly on the increase).

However, the various governments cannot agree – there is up to a 5-fold variation in the RDA figures for some nutrients from country to country. You may wonder which one is right.

Furthermore, what has not even begun to be established by government departments is the requirement for optimum – or tip-top – health. At most they will concede that children, pregnant and lactating women and the elderly have special nutrient needs. Luckily, however, there have been researchers interested in this area of health and we can look to them for information. One study, for instance, polled over 1000 doctors and their partners and showed that those who had an intake of 410 mg of vitamin C a day, more than 10 times the RDA, had the least signs of illness and the lowest incidence of colds – a comfort when you know that the average person has 3.5 colds per year!

Dr Emanuel Cheraskin, a leading nutrition researcher, and his colleagues at the University of Alabama, have provided some very interesting research leading to a new definition called SONAs (Suggested Optimum Nutrient Allowances). Their conclusion, after studying 13,500 people from 6 different areas of the USA, over a 15-year period, was that the healthiest people consistently had an intake of nutrients that were higher than the RDAs. They defined healthy individuals as those who not only showed a lack of deficiency disease, but who had the least clinical signs and symptoms of illnesses or degenerative diseases. They found that those individuals were eating a diet rich in nutrients relative to calories, and were frequently taking vitamin and mineral supplements. There are many scientific studies to back up the findings that intakes above the RDAs enhance resistance to infection, reduce the risk of degenerative diseases and help intellectual performance.

ARE VITAMIN SUPPLEMENTS NECESSARY?

I firmly believe that supplements are just that – supplementary to a good, varied diet. And I certainly would not ask someone to go against their principles if they felt very strongly that they did not want to give vitamin and mineral supplements to their child. Some people feel that it is like giving a child medicine and they would rather not do it. However, every time you use a formula milk it has been tailored nutritionally, with vitamins and minerals added or taken out. Many popular brands of cereals are enriched with nutrients – so, unwittingly, many of us are receiving supplements anyway. Guidelines recommend daily vitamin drops from the age of six months to five years. They also state that it may be advisable to give vitamin drops from the age of one month.

Refined foods, such as biscuits and white rice, deliver sufficient calories but not enough nutrients. Refined flour, for example, is stripped of around 90% of the minerals that you would get from wholemeal flour (though calcium is added back in) – it does not even have sufficient nutrients in it to support the life cycle of the common grain pest, the weevil! A vitamin and mineral supplement helps protect against these depleted foods. Also, if your child goes through a period of being picky about eating, a supplement will help to tide him over during this time. Even very mild anorexia (loss of appetite) has been linked to zinc deficiency, so it is worth some insurance.

It is not possible to give all the brand names of the various supplements and exclusion does not suggest that they are not as good as the ones listed, but I have listed some brands that I use successfully and that have child formulas (*see page 186*). If you follow the manufacturers' instructions they should be completely safe, although it is always possible to be sensitive to specific ingredients in particular brands. If this is the case switch brands. Remember that children have small livers and are therefore more sensitive to vitamin and mineral toxicity than adults, so it is important to get professional advice before embarking on a specialized programme. If your child has any particular health problems, see the relevant section in this book and consult your doctor or nutritionist.

I have included charts of vitamins and minerals and their uses and sources. Not all the nutrients have been covered, as it would read a bit like *War and Peace*, but all the main ones are included. It has not been possible to use the SONAs as the information is not available for such a young age group. However, the RDAs are available and this is the information given. SONAs are quite safely delivered by using a reputable, child-formula, vitamin and mineral drop or supplement.

💘 INSURANCE 💘

I always give my child a daily supplement as 'insurance' – insurance against the effects of pollution, agro-chemicals, nutrient-poor exhausted soil, depleted nutrient content of foods due to long-distance shipping, possible poor absorption of nutrients, and so on. It is a sad fact that analysis of the nutrient contents of fresh produce has shown that, compared to 50 years ago, there has been a 22% decline in mineral content. A daily multi-formula helps make up for this. I also always add a little extra vitamin C and some essential fats. I think that, in addition to a healthy diet, this is enough to keep most small children in tip-top health. In any event I prefer my child to be getting closer to the SONAs than the RDAs (*see opposite*) and a simple supplement programme helps to ensure this. Unless the product states otherwise, I would suggest giving any supplements with meals as they are better absorbed that way.

❦ VITAMINS – THEIR USES AND SOURCES ❦

VITAMIN	FEATURES	MAIN FUNCTIONS	FOOD SOURCES	AMOUNT minimum to prevent deficiency	
VITAMIN A	Fat soluble; excess causes toxicity; measured in micrograms (mcg) or in IUs (International Units)	Antioxidant; promotes eye health; protects against respiratory infections; promotes growth and healthy bones, teeth and gums; helps thyroid problems; protects vitamin C	Liver, cod-liver oil, egg yolks, full-fat dairy produce, herrings, mackerel	0 – 1yr 1 – 2 yr	350 mcg 400 mcg
BETA-CAROTENE	Water soluble; non-toxic; usually measured in mg (milligrams)	Converts to vitamin A; also has separate functions to vitamin A; antioxidant	Leafy green vegetables, carrots, sweet potatoes, cantaloupes, pumpkins	No recommended minimum	
VITAMIN B1 (also called thiamine)	Water soluble; easily destroyed by heat; non-toxic; measured in mg (milligrams)	Energy, carbohydrate digestion; used for nervous system, muscles, heart function; mental function, stress mechanism	Wholegrains, oatmeal, legumes, dried yeast, liver, pork, peanuts. Should be taken as part of B-complex if supplemented	0 – 6 mth 6 mth – 1 yr 1 – 2 yr	0.1 mg 0.4 mg 0.7 mg
VITAMIN B2 (also called riboflavin)	Water soluble; easily lost in cooking liquids; non-toxic; measured in mg (milligrams)	Promotes growth, healthy skin, hair and nails; helps metabolize carbohydrates, fats and proteins; energy production, stress handling; may be useful for sore mouth and lips	Green leafy vegetables, fish, yoghurt, liver, cottage cheese, milk. Should be taken as part of B-complex if supplemented	0 – 6 mth 6 mth – 1 yr 1 – 2 yr	0.4 mg 0.5 mg 0.8 mg
VITAMIN B3 (also known as niacin or nicotinic acid)	Member of B-complex family; water soluble; can be made in body from tryptophan amino acid; destroyed by food processing and leaching into water; non-toxic but high doses not recommended for children – may cause flushing; measured in mg (milligrams)	Essential for synthesis of sex hormones, thyroid hormone, insulin, cortisone and glucose tolerance factor; necessary for nervous system and brain function; needed for metabolism and energy; helps keep blood fats in balance	Lean meat, wheatgerm, figs, dates, avocados, fish, eggs, wholewheat, brewer's yeast; should be taken as part of B-complex if supplemented	0 – 6 mth 6 mth – 1 yr 1 – 2 yr	5 mg 6 mg 9 mg

VITAMIN	FEATURES	MAIN FUNCTIONS	FOOD SOURCES	AMOUNT minimum to prevent deficiency	
VITAMIN B5 (also known as pantothenic acid)	Water soluble; destroyed by food processing and heat; non-toxic; measured in mg (milligrams)	Vital for functioning of adrenal glands; required for conversion of fat and carbohydrates into energy; needed to manufacture antibodies; promotes wound healing; needed for mental function; reduces toxic effect of many antibodies (allergies)	Wholegrains, wheatgerm and bran, crude molasses, nuts, green vegetables, chicken, egg yolks, meat, liver. Should be taken as part of B-complex if supplemented	0 – 1 yr 1 – 2 yr	3 mg 5 mg
VITAMIN B6 (also called pyridoxine)	Water soluble; destroyed by long storage, food processing and high temperatures; non-toxic (excess in isolation could cause reversible neuropathy); measured in mg (milligrams)	Production of antibodies and red blood cells; needed to absorb vitamin B12; needed for all protein metabolism (i.e. growth, repair and enzymes); production of HCl (stomach acid) for protein digestion; works with zinc	Wheatgerm and bran, poultry, meat, liver, cantaloupes, cabbages, milk, blackstrap molasses, egg yolks, tuna, sardines, mackerel, leeks, kale, sprats, trout, salmon, cod. Should be taken as part of B-complex if supplemented	0 – 6 mth 6 mth – 1 yr 1 – 2 yr	0.5 mg 0.6 mg 1 mg
VITAMIN B12 (also called cobalamine)	Water soluble; destroyed by water, light and acids; often poorly absorbed; non-toxic; measured in mcg (micrograms)	Promotes growth; improves concentration and healthy nervous system; energy and fat, carbohydrate and protein metabolism; making red blood cells	Liver, beef, pork, fish, shellfish, eggs, milk, cheese; should be taken as part of B-complex if supplemented	0 – 6 mth 6 mth – 1 yr 1 – 2 yr	0.3 mcg 0.5 mcg 0.7 mcg
FOLIC ACID (also called folate or folacin)	Member of B-complex family; water soluble; destroyed by long-term storage; non-toxic; some children may have allergic skin reaction to it; measured in mcg (micrograms)	Needed for using proteins and carbo-hydrates; needed for antibody formation; helps ward off anaemia; protects against parasites and food poisoning; protects against neural tube defects early in pregnancy	Deep green leafy vegetables, carrots, egg yolks, apricots, pumpkins, beans, avocados, wholewheat and rye, cantaloupes	0 – 6 mth 6 mth – 1 yr 1 – 2 yr	25 mcg 35 mcg 50 mcg
BIOTIN	Member of B-complex family; water soluble; destroyed by food processing, antibiotics and lost in water; non-toxic; measured in mcg (micrograms)	Needed for metabolism of fats and proteins; maintains healthy skin, scalp and hair	Brewer's yeast, brown rice, nuts, fruit, egg yolks, beef liver. Should be taken as part of B-complex if supplemented	0 – 2 yr	150 mcg

VITAMIN	FEATURES	MAIN FUNCTIONS	FOOD SOURCES	AMOUNT minimum to prevent deficiency
CHOLINE	Member of B-complex family; a fat emulsifier; non-toxic; measured in mg (milligrams)	Able to go directly to brain, aids memory; controls cholesterol build-up; helps detoxification by eliminating toxins and drugs from liver	Green leafy vegetables, egg yolks, wheatgerm, liver, lecithin	No RDA
VITAMIN C (also known as ascorbic acid)	Water soluble; destroyed by heat, light, carbon monoxide (pollution) and aspirin; non-toxic (excess may cause diarrhoea); measured in mg (milligrams)	Health of immune system; anti-viral, anti-bacterial; skin, bone, cartilage formation and all connective tissue including gums and blood vessels; reduces histamine-type allergies; wound healing and post-surgery; may help prevent cot death; needed for stress management	Citrus fruit, strawberries, green leafy vegetables, cantaloupes, sweet peppers, cauliflowers, potatoes, sweet potatoes, kiwi fruit, bean sprouts, melons, jacket potatoes, spinach, broccoli, cabbages, turnips, liver	0–1yr 20–35 mg 1–2yr 40 mg
VITAMIN D (also known as calciferol)	Fat soluble; made by skin in sunlight; toxic in high doses; measured in micrograms (mcg) or IUs (International Units)	Co-factor for calcium and phosphorus in bone and teeth formation; works with vitamins A and C to help prevent colds	Sardines, herrings, salmon, tuna, egg yolks, fish oils, dairy produce	0–6 mth 8.5 mcg 7 mth–2 yr 7 mcg
VITAMIN E (also known as tocopherols)	Best form d-alpha-tocopherol; fat soluble; destroyed by heat, freezing, oxygen and food processing; non-toxic; measured in mg (milligrams) IUs (International Units)	Anti-oxidant; protects cell membranes; helps prevent scarring; anti-coagulant; protects against chlorinated water	Wheatgerm, vegetable oils (cold pressed, non-rancid), broccoli, Brussels sprouts, almonds, olive oil, eggs, spinach, soya beans, tomatoes, fresh nuts, carrots, sunflower seeds, wholegrain cereals including brown rice, oatmeal, rye and wholewheat crackers	no RDA but breast fed infants get 2.7 mg
VITAMIN K	Fat soluble; can be made by intestinal bacteria; destroyed by freezing, antibiotics and aspirin; not recommended in high doses; measured in micrograms (mcg)	Essential for blood-clotting agent, prothrombin; may be useful in bone metabolism	Yoghurt, alfalfa, egg yolks, safflower oil, kelp, fish-liver oils, leafy green vegetables, milk	0–2 yrs 10 mcg

❧ MINERALS – THEIR USES AND SOURCES ❧

MINERAL	FEATURES	MAIN FUNCTIONS	FOOD SOURCES	AMOUNT minimum to prevent deficiency
CALCIUM	Macro-mineral; works with magnesium, phosphorus and vitamin D; excess fats, oxalic acid (chocolate), phytic acid (grains) and phosphorus (cola drinks) are antagonistic; excess can lead to hypercalcaemia; measured in mg (milligrams)	Builds bones and teeth; used for blood clotting; essential for nerve message transmission; keeps heart beating regularly; helps usage of iron	Dairy produce, soya beans, sardines, salmon, peanuts, sunflower seeds, dried beans, green leafy vegetables, tofu, almonds, sesame seeds, broccoli	0–6 mth 350 mg 6 mth–2 yr 450 mg
CHROMIUM	Micro-mineral; no known toxicity; measured in micrograms (mcg)	Used for glucose tolerance factor to work with insulin and balance blood sugar levels; helps supply protein to where it is needed; helps to lower cholesterol levels; associated with longevity in trials	Shellfish, chicken, brewer's yeast, brown rice, rye bread, calves' liver, carrots, lettuces, eggs, bananas, cabbages, oranges, green beans, mushrooms, parsnips, apples, strawberries, potatoes, milk, butter	0–2 yr 10–60 mcg
IODINE	Micro-mineral; no known toxicity but excess may result in over-active thyroid; measured in micrograms (mcg)	Used by the thyroid gland to produce thyroxine hormone; thyroid hormone is needed for metabolism and proper mental function	Kelp, seaweed, all seafood, vegetables grown in iodine-rich soil, iodized salt	0–6 mth 40 mcg 6 mth–1 yr 50 mcg 1–2 yr 70 mcg
IRON (prefix 'ferric' often used on labels)	Micro-mineral; can be toxic in high amounts; vitamin C helps its absorption; measured in mg (milligrams)	Needed for red blood cell formation; used for energy production; needed to help metabolise B-vitamins	Liver, dried peaches, red meat, egg yolks, nuts, asparagus, oatmeal, blackstrap molasses, seaweed, parsley, figs, cherries, bananas, avocados, brown rice, potatoes, green peas, prunes, sunflower seeds, raisins, walnuts, mushrooms, kale, broccoli	0–6 mth 6 mg 6 mth–2 yr 10 mg

MINERAL	FEATURES	MAIN FUNCTIONS	FOOD SOURCES	AMOUNT minimum to prevent deficiency	
MAGNESIUM	Macro-mineral; can be toxic in excess; can be destroyed by some medicines; measured in mg (milligrams)	Needed for calcium metabolism; used for the stress response; needed for the energy cycle; essential for nerve and muscle function; important for mental function	All dark green vegetables (chlorophyll uses magnesium as we use iron for red blood cells), lemons, grapefruits, almonds, seeds, figs, yellow corn, aubergines, raisins, brazil nuts, carrots, mushrooms, crab, tomatoes, garlic, onions, chicken, potatoes	0 – 6 mth 6 mth – 1 yr 1 – 2 yr	40 mg 65 mg 80 mg
MANGANESE	Micro-mineral; toxicity rare; measured in mg (milligrams)	Important for bone structure; used in the energy cycle; needed for digestion; used by the thyroid gland	Nuts, green leafy vegetables, peas, beetroot, egg yolks, wholegrain cereals	0 – 6 mth 6 mth – 2 yr	0.3 – 0.6 mg 1.0 mg
SELENIUM	Micro-mineral; toxic in high doses; easily destroyed by food processing; measured in micrograms (mcg)	An important anti-oxidant; helps oxygen utilization; provides elasticity in tissues; makes vitamin E more effective	Wheatgerm and bran, tuna, tomatoes, broccoli, brazil nuts	0 – 6 mth 6 mth – 1 yr 1 – 2 yr	10 mcg 15 mcg 20 mcg
ZINC	Micro-mineral; can be toxic in very high doses; measured in mg (milligrams)	Needed for all protein metabolism including growth, cell repair and enzyme production; essential for reproductive organs	Meat, pumpkin seeds, sunflower seeds, wheatgerm, eggs, brewer's yeast, sardines, chicken, cucumbers, brazil nuts, egg yolks, carrots, oats, rye, cauliflowers, walnuts, almonds, buckwheat, lettuces, tuna, berries, brown rice	0 mth – 1 yr 1 – 2 yr	5 mg 10 mg

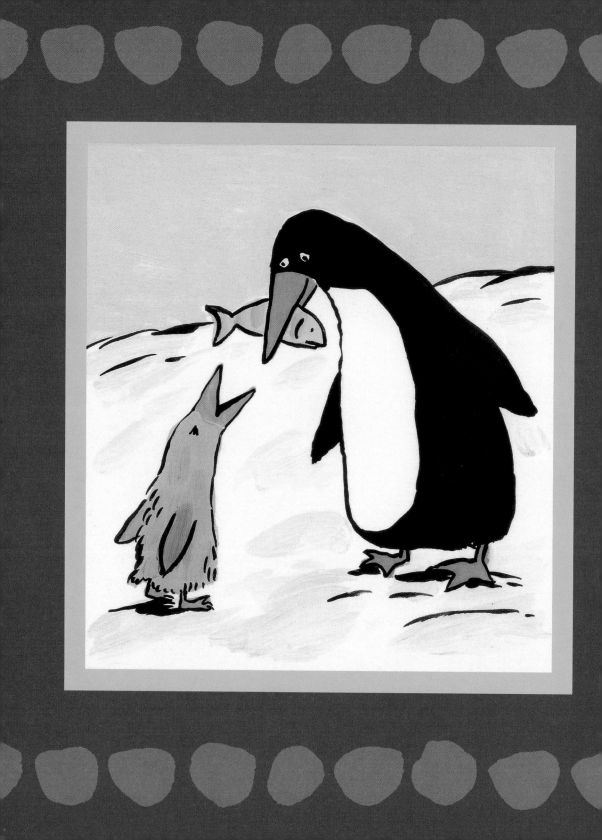

5

WHAT YOUR CHILD REALLY NEEDS

You will hear, time and time again, that you can get everything you need from a well-balanced diet. But what does that mean, and is it true? Is the same well-balanced diet appropriate for everyone? The people who are most likely to tell you this are those who have a limited training in nutrition. Sadly, this includes many doctors, whose surgeries may be full of people with every degenerative disease possible. The simple truth is that most people do not have what even approximates to a well-balanced diet. And those who do may still have problems, because of the poor nutrient levels in the food.

WHAT IS A WELL-BALANCED DIET?

The most common misconception is that if your child is getting sufficient macro-nutrients – proteins, fats and carbohydrates – and calories, he will automatically have a well-balanced diet and sufficient micro-nutrients such as zinc, chromium or selenium. This is not a foregone conclusion, and needs to be kept under constant review. You can do this by examining the quality of the proteins, fats and carbohydrates. Is sufficient protein coming from a vegetarian source? Are there enough of the essential fats in your child's diet? Are the carbohydrates coming principally from fibre-rich complex sources or from simple starches? The average calorie needs are around 800 calories a day for babies of 7–9 months, and 1200 calories for a toddler of 1–2 years. Please do remember that with calories it is not just the quantity, but also the quality that counts. Make sure the calories come from the wholefood sources suggested in this book, rather than refined and processed foods.

ALARMING STATISTICS

Study after study shows that the average child – not the undernourished child – gets less than the government recommended levels for a number of nutrients.

❧ THE AVERAGE DIET ❧

The average diet consists of (by calories):
* 40% fat
* 15% protein
* 45% carbohydrate – of which 25% is starch and 20% is sugar

Government guidelines state that the ideal diet should look like this (by calories):
* 30% fat – of which 10% is saturated and 20% unsaturated
* 15% protein
* 55% carbohydrate – of which 45% is complex carbohydrates and 10% is sugar

For children I would recommend that they have slightly more fat in their diet than this as they need extra calories in the early years (about 35%). The trick is to use the right fats (*see page 46*) and not to carry this high dietary fat content over into adulthood.

In simple terms this means that the ideal diet for a child should look like this (by food type):
* 70% vegetables, fruit, grains, beans, pulses and seeds
* 30% fish, meat, dairy products (or vegetarian / vegan equivalents) and added fats

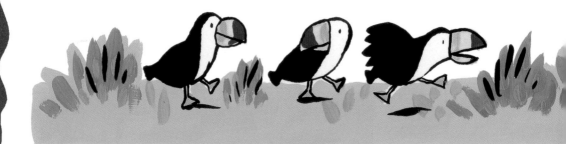

The most recent survey of the youngest of British children, aged one and a half to four and a half, has highlighted important areas that need to be addressed, not only by nutritionists, schools and educators, but also by parents.

This is the picture for small children today:

❦ Around three-quarters of children drank soft-drinks, and ate white bread, potato crisps and chocolate confectionery.

❦ At the same time raw vegetables and salads were eaten by less than a quarter of children, and leafy green vegetables were only eaten by around a third (and then only in small amounts).

❦ Peas, carrots and baked beans were the only vegetables to be eaten by the highest number of children – around 50 per cent.

❦ Only about a fifth of children eat the recommended five portions of fruit and vegetables daily.

❦ One fifth of calories are eaten away from the home (which often means higher salt, sugar and fat).

❦ Vitamin D intakes (important for bone health) average only one-sixth of the RNI for all children.

❦ Half of children have vitamin A intakes lower than the RNI (reference nutrient intake).

❦ Eighty-four per cent got less than the RNI for iron (important for mental development).

❦ Seventy-two per cent achieved less than the RNI for zinc (important for growth).

All the authorities, including the World Health Organization, recommend that we eat five portions of fruit and vegetables a day. Consumption of fruit and vegetables has gone down by 30% since 1970 and it has been remarked in studies that children often get the recommended amount only once a year – with their Christmas meal.

❦ VARIETY - THE SPICE OF LIFE ❦

Without a doubt, the most important message that I need to get across, and will repeat constantly, is that of variety. About 80% of our food intake comes from only 11 foods – variety is necessary to get the maximum range of nutrients.

To get the maximum number of vitamins and minerals, the two different types of fibre, phytonutrients (good plant chemicals and vitamin co-factors) and the right sort of fats, you need to encourage your child to have a broad range of tastes that allows for a varied diet. Having said this, please do not worry if your child goes through a phase of eating only sausages and beans. It happens all the time, and in the short term will do no harm. In the long term it pays to find a way out of this. Leading by example is obviously ideal; having a wide choice of foods at home is important, experimenting with the unfamiliar is critical and learning what constitutes variety is vital.

For instance, if you give your child wheat flakes and milk for breakfast, grilled cheese on wholemeal toast for lunch and pasta with a white sauce for the evening meal, you might think that you have offered a varied diet during the course of the day. You have, however, simply given wheat and dairy products at every sitting and almost no variety. Before you feel too bad, this is a very common diet for adults, and we quite often give our children what we eat because, not surprisingly, it is easier.

If you were to substitute porridge oats in the morning, tuna and tomato on toast for lunch and a rice and vegetable dish in the evening, you will have instantly broadened the variety to include at least two different grains, reduced the dependency on dairy and included a few vegetables in the day's diet. This is without making massive changes or making much extra effort.

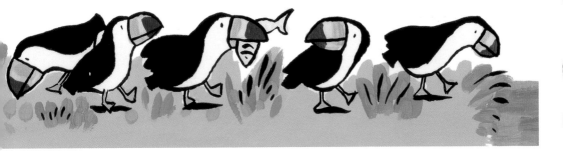

THE ENERGY
ROLLER-COASTER

It may seem strange to talk about maintaining good energy levels when discussing small children. Many parents are begging for mercy by the end of each day, as their child seems to have an endless supply of energy.

Whenever there is a problem with energy levels the culprit is most often an imbalance of blood sugar. It is a sad fact that this difficulty almost always starts in infancy.

We are designed to run, principally, on glucose as our source of fuel. Glucose is the end product of all our carbohydrate consumption, in whatever form it comes, refined or complex. It is transported to every cell in the body, including the brain which uses more than its fair share (30% of glucose) in relation to its weight (5% of body weight) – an indication of its importance. Adults have about two teaspoons of glucose in their blood at any one time; children will have a pro-rata amount depending on their size. When you compare this to the eight teaspoons of sugar in a candy bar you can see where there might be a dietary problem in relation to maintaining balanced blood sugar levels.

The important difference between refined and complex carbohydrates (*see page 48*) becomes obvious when you realize that problems start to happen when we get too quick a 'hit' of blood sugar – when it rises too quickly. This happens with refined carbohydrates, especially sugar – as in the candy bar above. Because high blood sugar is a dangerous situation which, if maintained, could lead to a diabetic coma, the body goes on red alert to lower the blood sugar and pours insulin into the system to do this. Insulin lowers blood sugar by storing the glucose in cells. If this roller-coaster goes on too often the insulin becomes trigger-happy and brings blood sugar down too low, too often. This is called a blood-sugar low. The quickest relief from this sugar low is to have another quick 'hit'.

This is why your child will nag for more juice or sweets at every opportunity. He is automatically doing what gives him quickest relief. Unfortunately, this also perpetuates the cycle and leads to a longer-term problem with blood sugar control.

Blood sugar balance will probably correct itself over time, or it can be avoided, by adhering to the guidelines that follow. One of the most important nutrients for blood sugar control is chromium,

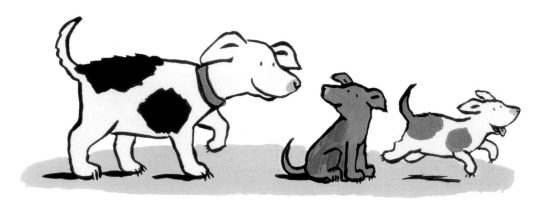

which is the core molecule for a substance that our bodies produce called glucose tolerance factor (GTF). GTF is produced by the liver and makes insulin more potent. Magnesium and vitamin B3 are also key nutrients in the sugar control mechanism. Chromium is found in whole grains, brewer's yeast, chicken and mushrooms; magnesium is found in green leafy vegetables, almonds and potatoes with their skins; vitamin B3 is found in avocados, fish, wheatgerm and dates (see page 53 for other sources of these nutrients).

MANAGING BLOOD SUGAR LEVELS

As I have already said, imbalanced blood sugar levels are the cause of more misery and symptoms in adults than almost any other health issue, and the problem starts in childhood. So, addressing this in your child's diet is a major step towards optimum health and an essential part of a balanced diet.

The way to avoid the problem in the first place, or to correct it if there is an existing problem is to:

- ❧ Provide small, frequent snacks to keep blood sugar levels constant. Breakfast should always be eaten though beware of some children's cereals which can be up to 50% sugar.
- ❧ Make sure meals and snacks consist of a good balance of complex carbohydrates (see page 48), proteins and fats. See page 103 for a list of suggested snacks.
- ❧ Avoid too much sugar, honey and sugary foods like cordials, candy, cake and biscuits. See the list on page 87 for hidden sugars.
- ❧ Avoid excessive use of fruit juices, or if you cannot avoid them make sure they are very diluted. Keep dried fruit to a reasonable minimum or mix them with protein and complex carbohydrate foods to add sweetness, but keeping the blood sugar effect in check. Fresh fruit is fine because the fibre in fruit helps to slow down the impact on blood sugar – juices do not have fibre.

❧ BLOOD SUGAR INDEX ❧

Here is a list of foods as they appear on the Blood Sugar (or Glycaemic) Index. This index charts different foods and the effect they have on blood sugar levels when compared to glucose, which has the most immediate effect and therefore scores 100 on the index. Generally speaking, it is wise to give your child foods that score below 60 on the scale and limit those that score between 61 and 100.

SUGARS:
Glucose 100
Honey, jam 87
White sugar 75
Milk chocolate 68
Dark chocolate 22
Fructose 20

FRUIT:
Watermelon 72
Raisins 64
Bananas 60
Grapes 60
Orange juice 46
Oranges 40
Apples 39
Apple juice 37

BREADS AND CRACKERS:
White bread 95
Rice cakes 82
French baguette 70

Brown bread 69
Oat cakes 54
Pumpernickel 40

GRAIN PRODUCTS:
White rice 72
Biscuits 70
White pasta 65
Pastry 59
Brown rice 50
Wholemeal pasta 42
Barley 22

CEREALS:
Puffed rice 90
Cornflakes 80
Wheat biscuits 75
Muesli 66
Porridge oats 49
Rice bran 19

PULSES:
Baked beans (sugar free) 40
Butter beans 36
Chickpeas 36
Haricot beans 31
Kidney beans 29
Lentils 29
Soya beans 15

DAIRY PRODUCTS:
Plain yoghurt 36
Whole milk 34
Skimmed milk 32

COOKED VEGETABLES:
Parsnips 97
Carrots 92
Potatoes 70
Beetroot 70
Yams .51
Sweet potatoes 48
Sweetcorn 48
Peas 40

VEGETARIAN
OR VEGAN CHILDREN

Studies consistently show that vegetarians and vegans have better heath ratings and lower incidences of degenerative diseases. I have to state my case and say here that neither my child nor I are vegetarian – We are mostly fishy-chicki-tarians, with a tiny amount of red meat from time to time. That is not to say that I do not acknowledge the obvious health benefits for most people of avoiding animal products if it is possible. Having said this, some adults and children do fare better with a little animal protein in their diets – we are all different.

Vegetarians avoid all animal flesh but, depending on their viewpoint, will eat eggs and/or dairy products. Vegans avoid all animal products.

From time to time there is a headline in the newspapers saying that children on a vegetarian diet exhibit some nutritional deficiencies and are less healthy than their meat-eating contemporaries. I suspect that this conflict arises because it is not enough simply to give up meat – there are many unhealthy vegetarians around. Simply giving up meat and living on a diet of chips, cheese sandwiches and processed vegetarian meals will not promote optimum health – and this way of eating is widespread. In nutrition circles these people are often called 'cheese-on-toast-vegetarians'. If you decide, for whatever reasons, that you would like your child to be a vegetarian or vegan, it is important to understand the issues and make relevant adjustments to their diet.

Variety becomes even more important as your child needs to get a wide range of nutrients. For instance, red meat is a very rich source of iron, zinc and vitamins B6 and B12. If meat is being eliminated – no bad thing in view of the accompanying levels of saturated fats and non-existent levels of fibre – you need to know which vegetarian food sources deliver these essential nutrients. See the list (opposite) for the richest supplemental food sources of nutrients. No vegetarian or vegan child should be without these.

The vegan diet may sound strange to some

people. However, most of us include many vegan meals in the 'normal' diet: baked beans on toast, mushrooms à la Grecque and gazpacho are all vegan dishes. It is true to say that studies of vegan groups have shown that, compared to vegetarians and meat eaters, vegan children tend to be slighter and a bit shorter. The reasons for this are unclear. It could be as a result of consuming fewer calories or lower levels of some nutrients or, even more sinister, it could conceivably be the lower amount of artificial growth hormones that vegan children ingest compared to those of us with meat and dairy in our diets.

❦ NUTRIENT WATCH ❦
• •
The main deficiency risks for vegetarians and vegans are likely to be the following:

Zinc and iron: Red meat is rich in these nutrients.

Vitamin B6: Zinc and B6 work together in the metabolism of proteins and tend to be found together in food sources.

Vitamin B12: A diet low in vitamin B1 and high in folic acid (such as a vegetarian diet) can mask a B12 deficiency. It can take up to five years to become apparent as all body stores of B12 have to be used up first.

Vegans are particularly at risk of B12 deficiency as current research is showing that the type of B12 that we get from animal sources is the only type that we can actually use. Vegans have traditionally used B12 supplements from sources such as spirulina; however it seems that the type of B12 that these provide is not readily used by the body.

Vitamin A: Infants do not convert beta-carotene derived from vegetable sources into vitamin A as well as adults. Sources of vitamin A are fatty, animal foods such as butter, egg yolks and liver as well as shellfish.

❧ VEGETARIAN AND VEGAN ❧ SOURCES OF NUTRIENTS

- Fresh, unroasted nuts including almonds, Brazil nuts, walnuts, pecans and hazel nuts are good sources of many nutrients including proteins, essential fats, calcium, magnesium and zinc. Nuts and seed should be ground.
- Fresh, unroasted seeds including sunflower, pumpkin and sesame seeds are good vegan sources of zinc, in addition to providing calcium, magnesium and essential fats.
- Vitamin B6 can be found in wheatgerm and bran, cantaloupes, cabbages and blackstrap molasses.
- Oatmeal, asparagus, brown rice, mushrooms, broccoli, kale, green peas, raisins and dried peaches are good vegan sources of iron.
- Vitamin C taken with vegetarian iron-rich meals will help to release and use the iron, since iron is not taken up from vegetable sources as easily as it is from meat. A small glass of orange juice should do the trick.
- Seaweed provides many of the trace elements to help metabolize the other nutrients more effectively and is a useful add-on for vegans in particular.
- Yeast extract and fortified cereals and soya milks provide vegan sources of vitamin B12.
- For vegetarians, eggs provide good amounts of zinc and iron.
- Peanuts are a good source of protein and peanut butter is popular with most children who do not have a peanut allergy. Not actually nuts, they are from the legume family, and because they grow underground (hence their other name, groundnuts) much of the world's crop is contaminated with aflatoxins which is a mycotoxin produced by mould. For this reason, I would limit their use (buying organic, sugar- and salt-free brands if you do use them) and concentrate on almond, pecan, cashew nut or sunflower seed butters available from health food shops. (*See page 96* for information on peanut allergies.)

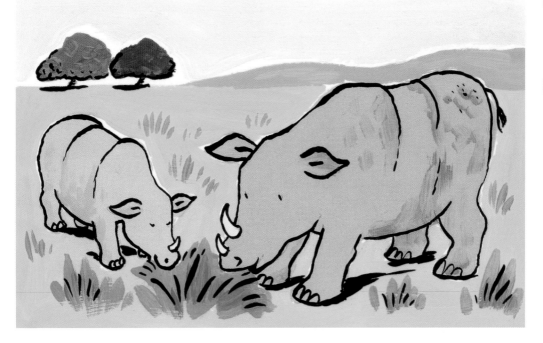

THE GREAT
DAIRY DEBATE

In the West, milk is taken for granted as an essential part of a small child's diet, even though many parts of the world do not use cow's milk at all. We are often told that a child will suffer without it and indeed, when most children are taken off the breast and put on to the bottle, or when weaned, they are usually put on to a form of cow's milk – either modified for bottle-feeding, or whole milk for older children. Government guidelines now definitely say that children should not be introduced to whole cow's milk until they are at least one year old.

A much advertised benefit of drinking milk for children is that it is a rich source of calcium and is therefore needed for growing bones and teeth. It has also been viewed as a good 'whole' food providing a balance of protein, fat and carbohydrate and a concentrated source of calories.

However, with the huge increase in childhood ailments, including asthma, eczema, glue ear and, alarmingly, childhood diabetes, more and more paediatricians are advising that milk, and dairy products in general, should be eliminated from children's diets. This is because dairy products have been closely implicated in all these problems in children who are dairy sensitive. This causes alarm among many parents who are concerned about

their children's dietary needs. Additionally, to confuse the issue further, many doctors and health visitors continue to encourage giving milk to toddlers and older children. Who is right?

I am firmly of the belief that dairy products are not needed for the human child and that, when consumed in excess, they cause more harm than good. It is true that some tolerate them perfectly well but if you suspect that milk does not agree with your child, you need to know what is involved in a dairy-free diet for your child.

BABY COWS

Cow's milk is really designed for baby cows, not baby humans. In fact human beings only introduced dairy foods into their diet around 10,000 years ago – around the time that man started to pen animals and grow crops. This means that, evolutionarily speaking, we are not really designed to consume milk. The casein, or protein, in cow's milk is very dense and hard to digest and does not compare at all well with human milk, for which we are designed. Even calves, when weaned, grow to maturity eating nothing but grass – they do not need milk to grow big and strong. Goat's milk is slightly more digestible for humans and, believe it or not, the closest milk to our own is donkey milk.

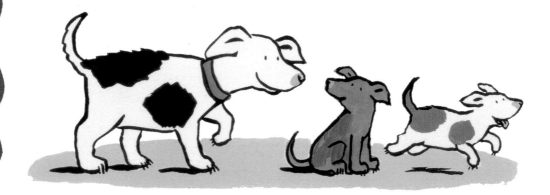

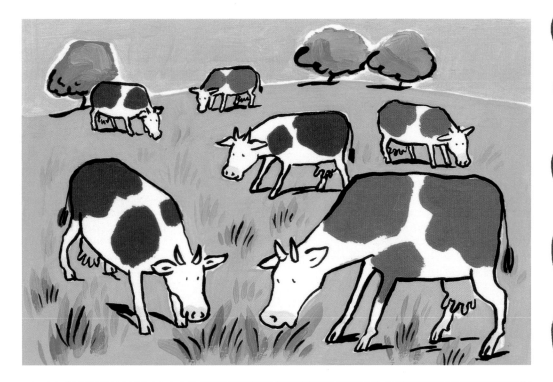

❧ WHY MILK IS PROBLEMATIC ❧

1 It is poorly digested, as discussed above. The casein coagulates into large clumps on contact with stomach acid, which in turn have to be broken down into digestible molecules.

2 It has been estimated that around seven per cent of babies have a cow's milk protein allergy, making it one of the most common allergens. Babies not exposed to cow's formula milk in the first six to nine months of life are less likely to develop this problem.

3 It can cause a problem in lactose-intolerant children who lack sufficient amounts of the milk sugar-digesting enzyme, lactase.

4 Dairy products are also known to be 'mucus forming', which can contribute to upper-respiratory tract infections and also to glue ear, both of which plague many small children.

5 Because it is rich in saturated animal fats, it favours a metabolic byproduct called arachadonic acid, which, in excess, is an inflammatory substance. It is therefore implicated in eczema and asthma, which are both inflammatory problems.

6 And finally, there is new research to show that the cow's milk protein may be a contributory factor triggering the onset of childhood, insulin-dependent, diabetes in genetically susceptible children. This type of diabetes, which used to be comparatively rare, has been increasing at a rate of 10% a year in children under five years of age. Researchers think that proteins in cow's milk may prompt the child's immune system to attack insulin-producing cells in the pancreas. This is still under review, but seems a serious possibility which may be substantiated with further research.

THE DAIRY
DOWNSIDES

If you have elected to avoid milk and dairy products the main concern is usually a reduced intake of calcium. However, calcium from milk is not particularly well utilized by the body since it is in too concentrated a form. For calcium to be used effectively it needs to be in the right balance with magnesium. Milk has almost no magnesium. The foods that have absolutely the right balance of calcium to magnesium, ensuring the best utilization by the body, are green leafy vegetables like cabbage and Brussels sprouts and nuts and seeds which can be ground up and mixed with your child's food. A good varied diet with a lot of fresh foods will almost certainly provide sufficient calcium, especially for a young child whose metabolism is geared to absorbing it well. If you are worried about calcium intake, refer to the chart opposite for non-dairy sources of calcium.

Interestingly, we absorb calcium from our diets according to our needs – healthy adults absorb around 20–30%. However in times of greater need, such as pregnancy or during childhood – both periods of bone formation – up to 75% of dietary calcium is absorbed. Our bodies have very clever mechanisms for regulating the absorption.

The high calorie content of milk and cheese is often spoken about as one of its benefits. However, I would suggest that these foods are too filling for small children, and so actually prevent them from having the appetite to eat from a wide range of food

❤ A SPECIAL WORD ABOUT ❤ YOGHURT

There is always the exception that proves the rule and yoghurt is the one in this case. Because the live bacteria used in the process of making the yoghurt has eaten the milk sugars and, largely, predigested a lot of the proteins, it is more easily digested. Many people who are milk intolerant find they can eat yoghurt. Another consideration is that the calcium in yoghurt is more 'bio-available' to us than that from other dairy sources, because of the presence of B-vitamins manufactured by the bacteria in the yoghurt.

I would always advise eating the live 'bio' type, preferably one that has no added fruit or flavourings. Adding the fruit in the manufacturing process usually diminishes the bacterial content. You can also find live yoghurts made from ewe's and goat's milk as well as soya yoghurts. Using all these types keeps the variety going and avoids establishing problems. Do not become overdependent on them however – one a day is maximum. They are delicious to use as toppings for fruit and desserts and mix very well into savoury dishes to create lovely creamy sauces.

that would be more beneficial as far as delivering the best and most complete range of nutrients.

As for milk being viewed as a complete food, this balance of protein, fat and carbohydrate can be achieved from a varied diet; and milk is, in my view, a poor second best to giving a child more beneficial nutrition including a good range of fruit, vegetables and useful fats in the diet. The argument may be valid if you are going to feed your child fast foods and snacks, but is not valid if you care in the least about your child's nutritional needs being met from a varied, wholefood diet.

People in many Eastern cultures avoid milk and dairy products and, as long as they are well nourished, they have no problems with bone formation. Indeed, in later years, they have very low incidence of problems with osteoporosis.

I have known many children, strapping tall ones at that, who generally avoid dairy products and as a result enjoy better health than the average child among their peers, with no ill effects. I feel fortunate that my child is one of them.

If you are going to give your child dairy products, the cheeses that are least likely to cause adverse symptoms are parmesan, cottage cheese and ewe's or goat's milk cheeses.

The recipes in this book are largely dairy free, to give an idea of how easy it is to keep dairy exposure to a minimum.

❧ NON-DAIRY ❧ SOURCES OF CALCIUM

This is a deliberately extensive list to show how diverse calcium is in our diet. We really do not need to have a hang-up about dairy sources of calcium. The recommended calcium intake for a small child is 350–450 mg daily.

FOOD SOURCE:	QUANTITY:	CALCIUM PROVIDED:
Canned sardines	1 small can	400 mg
Enriched flour	100 g/4 oz	200 mg
Canned pink salmon	1 small can	150 mg
Tofu (calcium enriched)	100 g/4 oz	150 mg
Enriched soya milk	100 ml/ 3½ fl oz	140 mg
Spinach, (cooked)	100 g/4 oz	75 mg
Broccoli	75 g/3 oz	75 mg
Almonds	25 g/1 oz	50 mg
Soya beans, (cooked)	75 g/3 oz	50 mg
Orange	1 medium	50 mg
Kidney beans, (cooked)	75 g/3 oz	50 mg
Blackberries	100 g/4 oz	35 mg
Leeks	50 g/2 oz	30 mg
Cabbage	50 g/2 oz	30 mg
Carrot	1 medium	25 mg
Dates and raisins	35 g/1½ oz	25 mg
Egg	1 large	25 mg
Wholewheat bread	1 slice	25 mg
Peanut butter	2 tbsp	25 mg
Apple	1 medium	20 mg
Green beans	50 g/2 oz	20 mg
Kiwi fruit	1 medium	20 mg
Sunflower seeds	15 g/½ oz	20 mg
Pumpkin seeds	10 g/⅓ oz	15 mg
Lentils (cooked)	55 g/2¼ oz	15 mg
Cauliflower	50 g/2 oz	15 mg
Pear	1 medium	10 mg
Cantaloupe	100 g/4 oz	10 mg

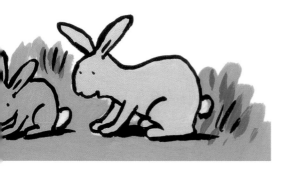

VOLUPTUOUS
VEGETABLES

When faced with parents who complain that their child just does not like vegetables, I cannot help wondering if, by serving the vegetables in a tasty way, they would have more success. Children love vegetables – just not all vegetables, all of the time. What they usually hate are bland, overcooked vegetables or ones with a bitter taste. The message is quite simple – good flavours will have children lapping up vegetables. Obviously it helps if you also eat and enjoy a wide range of vegetables. There are easy ways forward:

Sweet-tasting vegetables: These are sure-fire winners. For example red peppers, sweet potatoes, butternut squashes, peas, caramelized carrots, parsnips, sweetcorn, pumpkin and mangetout.
Hidden vegetables: Sneak them in. Finely chopped vegetables can be added to Spanish omelettes, savoury rice, tabbouleh, stuffed mushrooms, stuffed vine leaves or courgettes, for example.
A small grater: This is a great way to slip raw vegetables into your child's diet – grate some carrot, apple or cucumber and stir it into pureés, stews, soups or sauces.
Thick vegetable soups: If they are too thin, it is difficult to feed them to a small child. Try gazpacho,

borscht, minestrone, leek and potato or pumpkin. Stir in some yoghurt to make the soup extra creamy.
Go vegetarian: Try it for a meal or two a week. There are so many tasty vegetarian main courses to tickle your child's palate: mild vegetable curry, stir-fried vegetables and rice, bean stews or vegetarian shepherd's pie. The best sources of inspiration are ethnic cookbooks such as Indian, Chinese, Thai and Middle-Eastern, in addition to the recipes at the back of this book.
Sauces, purées and coulis: Another way to serve vegetables discreetly. Experiment with tomato sauces, or make sauces from puréed vegetables diluted with herb stock (*see Recipe Index*) or filtered water. This works especially well with carrots, broccoli, mushrooms and onions (*see Recipe Index*).
First course: Offer vegetables as a first course while your child is hungry.
Vegetarian meat alternatives: These are usually made from some combination of myco (mushroom) protein, soya and vegetables. Try sausages, nuggets and burgers – not as staples, but as reasonable standbys. They do not have all the advantages of fresh vegetables but neither do they have the disadvantages of meat – your child still gets the fibre.

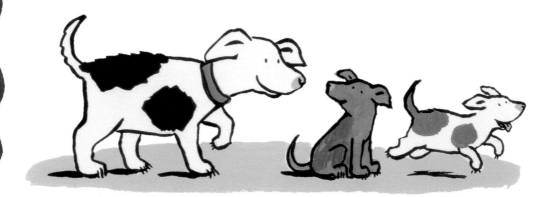

DRINKS
& LIQUIDS

Your child needs water. Many parents think that babies do not need it and that they get all the liquid necessary from breast or formula milk. In my view it is a good idea to develop a taste for water, and indeed a baby may cry because he is thirsty rather than hungry. Satisfying thirst with food (milk) can lead to a habit of mistaking the signals in later life. Water can be introduced after the first 10 weeks of bottle-feeding and breast-fed babies also benefit from water at this stage – it is particularly important in summer when dehydration is more of a risk. A baby may not take it at first, but persevere and he will. Nor will water fill up the stomach or dilute the digestive juices – it moves out of the stomach too quickly for that. Water should, of course, be boiled and then allowed to cool before giving to babies under six months of age and you should not use water from any questionable sources when travelling away from home.

I am unhappy with tap water as it often has some pollutants in it that the extraction process does not remove or that have leached into it from the conduit pipes. I would suggest using an inexpensive water filter. Alternatively, distilled or mineral waters are good options, but avoid giving a small child sparkling water

JUICES
There is no earthly reason why water should be sweetened with cordials or bottled fruit juices, with all the attendant problems for young teeth and sugar metabolism.

If you must flavour water, use freshly squeezed fruit diluted with water. It is worth buying a juicing machine and getting into the habit of making fresh juices of all descriptions as they are wonderfully rich in enzymes, vitamins and important phyto- (or plant-) chemicals. Shop-bought 'fresh' juices are very rarely truly fresh – it is amazing how the labelling laws allows this word to crop up. If the juice is truly freshly squeezed, and some supermarkets do provide fresh juices, then go for those – they cost

a little more but are worth it. Keep juices and fruit teas for mealtimes to minimise the sugar and acid impact on teeth. Between meals offer water.

❧ HELPFUL HERBS ❧
. . . .
A useful option is to make up herb teas and chill them ready for a thirsty young person. Mint tea (made by pouring boiling water over fresh mint leaves and then straining), lemon and ginger tea, vervain and camomile are just some of the options. You could also use some of the fruit teas that are widely available, have delicious aromas and have the enticing red colours of the cordials your child's friends may be drinking.

When weaning a child away from a taste for cordials, I have occasionally used a sweet-tasting powder called FOS (fructo-oligosaccharides), in moderation. It is an indigestible sugar, with no effect on blood sugar. It is also a good source of fibre and a growing medium for the good bowel bacteria, thus improving digestive health. Half a teaspoonful of FOS in a bottle or cup tastes very sweet, has nutritional advantages and can be used to reduce the dependency on sugary drinks over time. It is advised that children can use FOS after they have been weaned. Because FOS is a similar compound to inulin found in the renowned windy vegetable, Jerusalem artichokes, it may result in some wind in some children. Most do not have a problem with it, but be aware that this a possibility. See the addresses on page 186 for suppliers.

Incidentally, I made an interesting discovery when my child was reaching for his friends' cordial cartons on a regular basis and I was a bit fed up that all my good groundwork seemed to be for nothing. Eventually I guessed that it was actually the straws that he wanted. I started carrying around a straw for him to use and that was the end of the problem.

LIVE FOOD
THE LIFE FORCE

In the 400,000 years since Homo sapiens evolved on the planet, and for the majority of the 45,000 years since anatomically modern man appeared, we did not cook or process our foods in any way. We were hunter-gatherers, which means we ate what we could kill or gather, and we would store only a few foods. We started cooking our food in what, in evolutionary terms, is the twinkling of an eye.

Of course, the biggest revolution in food supply has come in the last 200 years with intensive farming, refrigeration and, more recently, with the advent of supermarkets providing easy access to foods from around the globe.

In terms of what we have on our plates, the most important change is the amount of cooked and processed food that we eat. And, of course, cooking is a form of processing. When you apply heat to a food you automatically change its molecular structure. This renders it less useful to our bodies, which developed for a different type of food availability. The changes in our eating habits have been too fast and too radical for evolution to catch up with. From a safety point of view it is important to cook many foods for children properly, to avoid problems with contamination by bacteria and parasites. This is why we have pasteurized milk and why it is advised not to give unpasteurized cheeses to children or pregnant women. It is also important to cook meat thoroughly for the same reason. For practical reasons we also need to cook foods that cannot be eaten raw, such as potatoes and pulses. It is also true that some compounds, carotenes in particular from foods like tomatoes and carrots, are more absorbable from cooked foods.

However, the more raw fruit, vegetables and sprouted seeds that can be obtained in the diet, the better. They are a rich source of vitamins, minerals, fibre, water and enzymes. Cooked food can be viewed as 'dead' food and raw food as 'live' food. This might be a bit extreme, obviously we get something from cooked food and we need to seek a balance. In her book, *Raw Energy* (*see page 186*),

Leslie Kenton refers to the fact that cooked foods were termed by Professor Werner Kollath at the University of Rostock in the 1950s as foods that provided 'meso-health' – adequate to sustain life but likely to lead, in the long term, to degenerative diseases.

❦ COOKED FOOD ❦

Obviously cooked food tastes good, but it is useful to know that when you do cook food you do the following:

❦ Change the protein structure.

❦ Change the nature of the unsaturated fats.

❦ Destroy some of the vitamins.

❦ Lose minerals to any cooking water.

❦ In some cases, turn complex carbohydrates into simple carbohydrates (for example when brown rice is overcooked).

❦ Create carcinogenic compounds by browning or crisping (burning) foods.

❦ Destroy the enzymes that are helpful to digestion. (For instance, raw milk comes with lactase enzymes, raw meat with protease enzymes, raw fat comes with lipase enzymes, and so on. The idea of raw food of this type may sound revolting, but for example with Japanese sushi – which some of us enjoy – you get the meat- and fat-digesting enzymes with the food.

PHYTONUTRIENTS

There is a whole new area of research, focusing on what are termed 'phytonutrients'. Another name for these is 'nutriceuticals' – as opposed to pharmaceuticals. This is the study of plant compounds, or chemicals, and their applications for therapeutic use and they are now coming into the domain of high-tech research. The interest does not centre on the known essential nutrients – vitamins and minerals – but on the thousands of non-essential compounds that seem to have enormously beneficial effects on human physiology.

Also of interest is the synergistic aspect to their functioning – how they work together so that the whole is more than the component parts. This is one of the big differences between nutritional and drug therapy. Drug therapy isolates single compounds and concentrates them, despite the fact that this usually has a downside – you need only read the long lists of side effects and contra-indications for most drugs to know this. Phytonutrients, however, although isolated for study purposes, are provided with the enhancing factors that the plant provides in nature when eaten as a whole, and usually raw, plant. For example, beta-carotene is a major component of carrots, but carrots also provide a wide range of carotenides to support the beta-carotene.

Luckily you do not need to be at the cutting edge of research to feel the benefits of all these phytonutrients. You and your child simply need to eat a good amount of raw food in your diet. The message here is that raw food can, and does, act as an enhancer of good health, and has potent protective properties against disease.

THE POWER IS IN THE SEED

Nutritionally speaking, any 'potential plant' is the most concentrated source of nutrients. These nutrients have been concentrated for the tremendous growth spurt, into a plant, that is anticipated. We can take advantage of that intense source of nutrients – be it from seeds, grains, beans, pulses, fruit or roots.

A super high-charged, power-packed source of nutrients is provided by sprouting beans, pulses, seeds and grains. When sprouted they actually increase their nutrient content by between 200 and 2000% with the simple addition of water.

Sprouting also neutralizes some of the factors that make them less digestible and, in some cases, slightly toxic. It gets rid of the trypsin inhibitors and phytic acid that are in the unsprouted germ. They are simplicity itself to sprout at home and older children love to do this as a project. Toddlers adore them as they can be picked up easily with little fingers and taste really sweet. They can be sprinkled on dishes to boost the nutrient content of any meal.

❦ POWER PACKED ❦

Grains, seeds and pulses, when sprouted, increase their levels of nutrients. For example, sprouted oats multiply their nutrient content as follows:

NUTRIENT:	% OF INCREASE:
Vitamin B2	2000%
Biotin	50%
Vitamin B5	200%
Vitamin B6	500%
Folic acid	600%
Vitamin C	600%

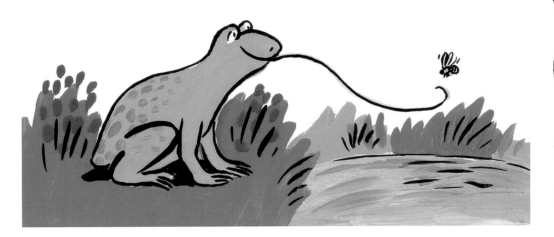

RAW FOOD
EASY IDEAS

Including some raw food at most meals is a worthwhile exercise providing valuable nutrients and enzymes. It is quite easy to introduce more raw food into your child's diet with a little forethought. Below are a few suggestions.

Finger foods: Carrot, cucumber, celery (strings removed) or red and yellow pepper sticks; mangetout and raw sweet peas; chunks of avocado; fruit chunks or fruit salad; cherry tomatoes; florets of cauliflower and broccoli; slices of mushrooms or radishes – all of these make good foods for little fingers.

Juices: Raw fruit and vegetable mixtures make ideal drinks. Try carrot and apple, tomato and cucumber, watermelon and beetroot or pear and celery.

Raw soups: Gazpacho, raw cucumber soup, raw tomato soup and raw borscht are good examples.

Finely chopped salads: Tabbouleh, tomato and onion salad and coleslaw are good options. Or make a rainbow salad: place grated carrot, beetroot and cucumber in separate little mounds and sprinkle with lemon juice and a little walnut oil if you wish.

Hummus: Try making this with sprouted chickpeas instead of cooked ones (*see Recipe Index*).

Coulis and shakes: Many fruit are suitable; try mango, peach, papaya, pineapple, banana, blackcurrant or raspberry – the last two for those over six months old only, because of the seeds.

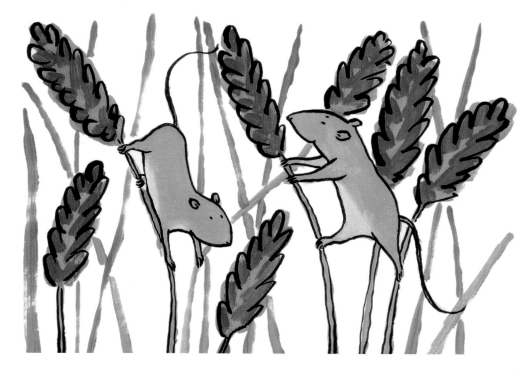

Make the shakes with soya, rice or oat milk if you want to avoid dairy products. For a coulis, simply whisk up the fruit in a blender to serve as a delicious fruity sauce.

Ground fresh seeds and nuts: Pumpkin and sunflower seeds or pine kernels, finely ground in a clean coffee grinder, have a nutty taste and can be sprinkled on anything – from vegetables to soups to salads. Beware if you think your child may have an allergy (*see page 96*).

Grating and snipping: The raw food content of a cooked meal can be boosted by grating carrots, apples or cucumbers; by finely chopping spring onions, or by using kitchen scissors to snip bean sprouts, chives or herbs. A hand-held food mill (mouli) can be used to finely shred raw mushrooms, onions and most other vegetables; or use a fork to mash some skinned tomatoes.

Fresh herbs: For the last 2000 years, herbs have been used for a range of medicinal uses and have a range of protective plant compounds. At every opportunity you can use a mouli, grinder or scissors to chop herbs into your baby's food. Fresh herbs to experiment with include parsley, chives, dill, mint, basil, coriander, tarragon, thyme and oregano.

❧ HOW TO SPROUT BEANS, PULSES, ❧ SEEDS AND GRAINS

Stock up on the following equipment: a large, see-through, wide-necked glass jar or bowl; cheesecloth or a tea towel and a large rubber band to secure it; a strainer; a water filter; a warm place such as an airing cupboard; a household plant water sprayer.

What can be sprouted? Mung beans, chickpeas, whole lentils, oat grains, sunflower seeds, pumpkin seeds, alfalfa, mustard seeds, sesame seeds, aduki beans, soya beans, wheat grains, rye grains, barley and millet. The method is the same for all, although the sprouting times are different for each. Here, beans are referred to throughout for simplicity.

❧ First clean the beans, removing any stones, broken beans or dirt. Rinse well under running water. You do not need too many beans since, when they sprout, they increase in volume by quite a lot. Experiment with quantities for your needs – it is cheap to do so since the basic ingredients are so inexpensive.

❧ Put the beans into your container and make sure they are covered with water to soak. It is best to use filtered, mineral or boiled water for this as they will absorb quite a lot of the water and some beans do not sprout well with plain tap water because of the chlorine content.

❧ Cover and leave the beans to soak overnight in a warm, dark place.

❧ The next day, discard the soaking water. If there is no water left give the beans a bit more to absorb and leave for a few hours more.

❧ Tip the beans into a sieve and rinse well under running water. Put them back in the jar. Make sure they are well drained, as excess water at this stage may make them rot. Cover again and put them back in the warm, and preferably dark, place.

❧ Repeat the rinsing and soaking at night and in the morning. After three to five days you will have lots of lovely sprouts and you can now put them on the windowsill to catch the sunlight. Spray them with water from a plant sprayer. They will be ready to eat within the next five to twenty-four hours, when the leaves are turning green. If you want to get rid of the hulls, place them in a bowl of water and stir them around – the hulls will float to the top.

❧ They can be stored in the refrigerator in an airtight container or a plastic bag for a couple of days. If you are really keen on sprouting you can get a rota going, with different types of sprouts, so that you are never without. For those seeking a more convenient option, many health food shops and supermarkets now sell bean sprouts and sprouted seeds.

WONDER
FOODS

Some foods are recognized as providing super-charged nutrition and protection from degenerative diseases. They are incredibly valuable to include in the diet. If possible, I would aim to give to your child the 'wonder foods' below at least once a week, when you have introduced them to a complete variety of foods. It is still important to achieve a wide variety of foods in your child's diet – just make sure he has his fair share of the wonder foods. The meal-planner for 15–24 Months on page 158 illustrates how easily this can be done.

This list is not exhaustive and the fact, for example, that strawberries, watercress and lentils have been left out does not mean that they are not also power-packed foods. The following, however, have particularly interesting properties that are worth knowing about.

APPLES
It is tempting to say 'An apple a day keeps the doctor away' – and I have succumbed. A rich source of vitamin C, apples also have high levels of pectin. These help to keep cholesterol levels stable and studies have shown that, in adults, two apples a day reduce cholesterol levels by 10%. Pectin is a powerful detoxifier and binds to heavy metals such as lead and mercury in the body and then carries them out when excreted. Apples also contain malic and tartaric acid, which help to neutralize the acid byproducts of digestion, helping to cope with excess proteins and fats. They can easily be grated into a variety of dishes.

APRICOTS
Along with other orange-coloured foods – cantaloupes, squashes, pumpkins and yellow peppers – apricots are very rich in antioxidants, in particular beta-carotene and the rest of the carotenoids. They are highly protective against infections, particularly infections of the respiratory system. Apricots are also high in iron. They are delicious as an accompaniment to both sweet and savoury dishes.

BROCCOLI
Together with other members of the cruciferous family – cabbages, kale, cauliflowers, Brussels sprouts, radishes, turnips and watercress – broccoli is well established as a potent weapon in the fight against cancer. Studies at the US National Cancer Institute directly correlated high intake of these vegetables to reduced risk. Compounds that have been shown to be active in broccoli and other crucifers include indols and carotenoids. New research into the glucosinolates they contain shows that they break down into sulphoraphane in the body, which has a powerful anticancer effect. Broccoli is also a good source of iron. Raw broccoli and cauliflower florets make good crudités for dips, or add to vegetable soups and stews. Broccoli is delicious Chinese style, stir-fried with sesame oil and soya sauce.

BROWN RICE
This contains a compound called gamma-oryzanol, which has remarkable properties in keeping the digestive tract healthy and helping to normalize the production of gastric juices. Unpolished, wholegrain rice also provides a rich variety of nutrients including iron, magnesium, vitamin E and vitamin B6. Brown rice is particularly good for keeping blood sugar levels constant and is often used in hypoallergenic diets as it is so well tolerated by most people. (*See the Recipe Index for ideas*).

CABBAGES
Apart from all the benefits described above for broccoli, cabbage also produces a substance called, imaginatively, cabagin – also known as vitamin U. Cabbages protect against developing disturbances of the digestive tract. They are rich in vitamin C, iron and also magnesium from their high chlorophyll content. They may also provide good

❦ FLAX OIL ❦

This is derived from the linseed, but called flax oil in order to differentiate it from the linseed oil used for restoring furniture. To prevent damaging rancidity, flax oil must be cold pressed and bought in small quantities, in dark glass bottles and kept refrigerated. It is rich in both of the essential fats, omega-3 and omega-6, which are so important for the functioning of every cell in the body. It can help to keep allergies at bay, keeps the skin smooth and supple, is important for nerve and brain structure and also for hormone production. Flax oil must not be heated, but can be added to salads, or stirred into warm (but not hot) cereals, vegetables and soups. A teaspoonful or two is sufficient for small children.

protection against radiation damage. A home-made coleslaw (*see Recipe Index*) provides raw cabbage, which is more protective than its overboiled counterpart. Sauerkraut, made from cabbage, ferments to produce lactic acid, which is cleansing for the digestive tract and helps to keep the bacterial contents of the bowels in good balance.

CARROTS

One carrot will supply enough beta-carotene to meet an adult's daily vitamin A requirement. Rich in the whole carotenoid family, carrots are also effective in supporting the immune system, helping with respiratory infections, maintaining skin integrity and are important for eye function. Carrots have been shown to be protective against certain cancers as they are rich in the antioxidants, including vitamins C and E. Carrot sticks are good snacks and grated raw carrot can be stirred into a variety of main meals.

GAME

Red meat is an important source of iron, zinc, vitamins B6 and B12. The problem with red meat is that it is also incredibly high in the saturated fats that are implicated in cancer, heart disease and all inflammatory diseases, including eczema, asthma, psoriasis and arthritis. The advantage of game meat is that it is, by definition, free-range and, because the animal's diet is completely different to the feed given to factory farm-raised animals, the fats in game meat are also completely different. Less than four per cent of their total weight are saturated fats. Because it is free-range game is also free of the chemicals, including large amounts of antibiotics and growth hormones, found in the meat of factory-farmed animals. At the risk of upsetting the faint-hearted, it is worth mentioning that it is very important to remove any lead shot that may remain in the meat. Game substitutes well for any red meat recipe.

GARLIC AND ONIONS

Garlic has been the subject of extensive research to discover the reasons for its superlative reputation as a cure-all in the folk medicine of a wide number of different cultures. It has well-established antiviral, antifungal and antibacterial properties. It has been shown to be effective against lung infections, urinary tract infections, arthritis and even heart disease and cancer. The active compounds allicin and alliin are the source of the strong-smelling parts. Garlic is also high in

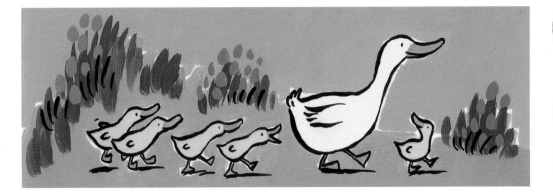

germanium, which actively promotes the uptake of oxygen at a cellular level, increasing its therapeutic benefit.

The onion shares most of the same attributes as garlic, and has a few of its own: it is helpful with asthma, anaemia and arthritis, and it lowers blood sugar levels. Garlic and onions are both rich in the sulphur amino acids that help detoxify heavy metal build-up in the body. In fact the whole onion family, including chives, spring onions and shallots, have similar benefits.

GRAPES

Grapes are the usual gift for invalids – with good reason. They have potent cleansing properties and are useful for a number of ailments, including anaemia, arthritis, gout and rheumatism. They seem to be regenerative for fatigue and convalescence from illness. They are regularly used by naturopaths for urinary, skin and inflammatory conditions. Since grapes tend to be excessively sprayed with chemicals it is advisable to wash them particularly well. Put a little vinegar in the washing water to help dislodge the waxy chemicals, and rinse well afterwards.

MOLASSES

This is the residue left when sugar is refined. Crude black molasses is very rich in the B-vitamins, potassium and iron. It even provides more calcium than milk! As with any refined food, sugar has had all the nutrients that are usually needed to metabolize it stripped away – this extract gives you what has been taken out of white sugar. Molasses is still a high-sugar food and should only be used sparingly in cooking and on cereals. It has a very distinctive taste that may take some getting used to.

MUSHROOMS

These are a valuable source of vegetable-based proteins and are also good sources of vitamins and minerals. The more exotic mushrooms, shiitake, maitake and reishi for example, have been researched a great deal to show that they offer various health benefits including being antiviral, cholesterol lowering, antiallergy, antioxidant, antibacterial and supporting the immune system. Mushrooms, finely chopped in a small food processor with some parsley, can be added to many dishes such as rice and other grains, minced meat stuffing and tomato sauce.

OATS

Whole oats have a particularly good reputation for having a positive influence on health. They are one of the only foods that are allowed to make health claims on packaging as they have been shown to lower cholesterol levels and other blood fats. They also help stabilize blood sugar levels, and are rich in a form of soluble fibre which protects intestinal and stomach surfaces. Oats also provide polyunsaturated fats, vitamin E, good amounts of the B-vitamins, calcium, magnesium, potassium and silicon, making them very useful for bones and teeth. Old-fashioned porridge oats are the best to eat, as the 'ready' versions are processed and provide less of these benefits. As well as making porridge you can also use oats for crunchy, sweet or savoury toppings (*see Recipe Index*).

OILY FISH

Oily fish include mackerel, sardines, salmon, pilchards, pink trout, tuna, anchovies, herrings and shark. They provide the omega-3 fats, DHA (docosahexanoic acid), which is used for building brain and nervous tissue, and EPA (eicosapentanoic acid) which is beneficial for cardiovascular health and inflammatory problems such as arthritis and skin diseases. Canned fish such as sardines still provide these oils but canned tuna is not a good source.

OLIVE OIL

This, a staple of the Mediterranean diet, has been the subject of much research which shows that it gives protection against heart disease and cancers. Olive oil is very high in the antioxidants, particularly vitamin E, and a range of phyto-nutrients with antioxidant properties. It has also been shown to help peristalsis (the squeezing motion) of the digestive tract so that it aids digestion and helps to remedy constipation. Olive oil should ideally be used in the cold-pressed 'extra-virgin' form since this is highest in these health-promoting substances.

PAPAYAS AND PINEAPPLES

These delicious tropical fruit are rich in enzymes that are useful for digestion when eaten fresh. The enzymes they contain are papain and bromelin and they break down proteins extremely effectively. Astoundingly, bromelin breaks down up to 1000 times its own weight of protein. It also helps to redress the body's acid/alkaline balance. They both help to clean up dead tissue in the gut wall, contributing to intestinal health. When they are in season this duo is a must.

SEAWEEDS

These sea vegetables are a valuable source of iodine, which is needed for good functioning of the thyroid gland. They are also rich in vitamin K, chlorophyll and alginic acid, a detoxifier, and deliver a wide range of ultra-trace minerals that our bodies require in minute quantities, but are important for maximum vitality. The easiest way to get a child to take a little is to use the Nori flakes or powdered seaweeds. They can be used as a salty-tasting condiment, and have a mild, herby flavour that is delicious with most savoury dishes.

SEEDS

Sunflower, pumpkin and sesame seeds and pine kernels are all little powerhouses of nutrition – the seeds concentrate vitamins and minerals for the benefit of the potential plant, making them an ideal snack for us. They are rich in the omega-6 series of essential fats, and pumpkin seeds are also a good source of the omega-3 series. They offer good amounts of zinc, magnesium and calcium. Seeds should be eaten fresh, not roasted, and bought in small quantities so they do not go rancid. For small children (*see also page 98*) they can all be ground into a fine nutty tasting powder to sprinkle on to savoury or sweet dishes – and, in fact, more of the nutrients are absorbed by doing this.

SPROUTED SEEDS, BEANS AND GRAINS

These can be made easily at home (*see page 75*). Sprouts are the germinated 'seed potential' and at the point when they have sprouted they are packed with more nutrients than either before or after. They are rich in plant enzymes, which enhance our own enzyme potential. Sprouts are probably the perfect food. They can be sprinkled on many dishes for a little extra 'crunch' or are great in a bowl as nibbles.

YOGHURT

I am talking here about plain, live or 'bio' yoghurt and not the sugary fruit yoghurts ('bio' or otherwise) that are poor relatives. Live yoghurt is rich in bacteria such as Lactobacillus bulgaricus, Lactobacillus acidophilus, Bifidus bifidum, Streptococcus thermophilus and other strains, which help to maintain the bacterial balance in the gut. The reason that yoghurt is easy to digest compared to milk is that the bacteria has predigested a lot of the milk proteins and milk sugars which cause problems in so many people. Some people with dairy allergies may still have a problem and can try ewe's milk, goat's milk or soya yoghurt. Most people, however, can safely eat this wonder food. Yoghurt makes a delicious topping for fruit and other desserts, can be used as an alternative to mayonnaise or can be stirred into savoury dishes at the last minute to make a creamy sauce.

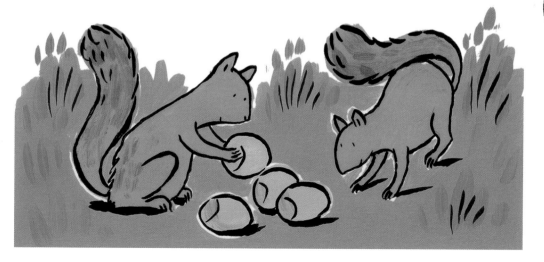

ORGANIC
FOODS

We have the luxury, these days, of a plentiful food supply. Walk into any supermarket or fruit and vegetable shop and you will see a massive array of plump, colourful, juicy produce. Much of it is available out of season, brought in from countries that have different growing seasons. All this may seem like a good thing – but what is lurking beneath the surface?

In order to provide this fine-looking produce, farming methods have been tailored to benefit the appearance of fruit and vegetables, frequently at the expense of the flavour and nutrient content. There is extensive use of pesticides and artificial fertilizers; some crops are sprayed many times with cocktails of many chemicals. These chemicals do not simply lie on the surface because the produce has been sprayed from the moment it is a seed or a tiny fruit, and the chemical becomes intrinsic to the flesh. Most of the chemicals do lie just beneath the surface and, despite it being a shame to have to peel fruit and vegetables, since most of the nutrients are just under the skin, it is a good idea to do so. Fruit and vegetables that are imported can have suspect vitamin levels as they have often been picked 'green' and then ripened in transit – sometimes artificially with gases. The storage and transit time itself, an average of three weeks from tree to shop, is not conducive to maintaining good nutrient levels. Imported produce hides another potential hazard since chemicals that are banned in Europe and the USA are often used in other countries, for example

DDT, although banned in the developed world, is still used for spraying produce in some Third World countries.

Many people seriously consider organic fruit and vegetables for the above reasons, but are then put off by higher prices, smaller fruit and vegetables, limited availability due to shorter growing seasons, less attractive produce and, the final insult, having to share their lettuce with the occasional worm. Frequently, they complain that organic produce goes off quicker than the produce they are used to.

IS IT WORTH THE EFFORT?

In my view the answer is a resounding yes! The distribution and availability of organic produce has improved immeasurably in the last few years as consumer demand grows. This means that prices are beginning to come down. I believe it is worth paying slightly more to ensure a chemical-free diet – our livers have enough problems dealing with other forms of pollution without adding agrochemicals to the soup. I like eating 'in season', and it is quite pleasing to get a few surprises in the box that is delivered weekly by my supplier – it stretches my culinary efforts. The produce may look slightly less appealing, but the acid test is the taste. When you eat tomatoes that actually taste of tomatoes rather than flavourless pulp, and spinach that is sweet, not bitter, it all seems well worth it.

The main concern has to be nutrient levels in foods. The old research methods found little

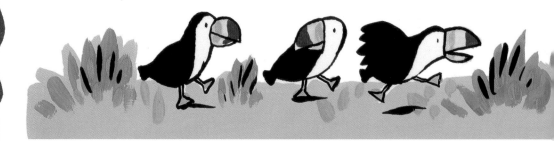

difference between organic and non-organic. However, modern research shows that organic foods have, on average, twice the nutrient levels of commercial produce. On a final note, sharing my produce with the occasional bug tells me that, if it is good enough for them to eat, then it must be all right for me and my child – bugs are a lot pickier than human beings, it would appear.

Now to the question of meat and milk. Factory-farmed animals, including fish, are subject to a completely different diet from one that they would have in the wild. On the basis that they are what they eat, just as much as humans, this means that their composition, especially their fatty composition, is far from ideal. Our ancestors, who lived on hunted meat, had a proportion of the essential fats in their diet coming from meat – this is no longer the case and farmed meat now mostly provides saturated fats.

Depending on where factory-farmed animals are reared, they are likely to contain hormones, including growth hormones, agro-chemicals from feed and antibiotics. It has been estimated that around 50% of the antibiotics that we consume come not from the doctor, but from the meat, dairy and egg products that we eat since they are used as growth promoters. The implications of the high amounts of antibiotics that we consume, in terms of disease resistance and digestive tract health, are enormous. Real free-range game avoids most of these problems and provides some of the good essential fats.

It is also interesting to note that organically reared animals become more fertile over three generations – in stark contrast to what is happening among the human population, which is suffering a fall in fertility. Organic meat and dairy produce is readily available: most major supermarkets carry some items and home delivery is easy to arrange. It is a little more expensive but if, as I suggest, you cut back slightly on meat consumption and increase vegetable consumption, then most budgets will feel the pinch less – it is worth it. (*see page 187* for lists of suppliers.)

❦ LIVER ❦

Liver really is a tremendous food as it is densely packed with so many nutrients. The reason for this is that the liver is the organ in which nutrients are stored for the animal's benefit. Liver is rich in vitamins A, B complex and K (pork liver) and the minerals iron, chromium, cobalt, copper, selenium and zinc – it is a bit like taking a supplement! The liver also has many other functions, and one of its most important jobs is to detoxify chemicals. Sadly, this means that in addition to it being a storehouse for nutrients, it is also loaded up with pollutants. All the agro-chemicals that are sprayed on the grass that the animal eats and all the antibiotics and growth enhancers that are put into the animal's feed or water will have to go through the liver. So what do you do?

If you do not buy any other organic food, do make sure that you buy organic liver because, in my view, it is unsafe to give small children liver from any other source. And this is a great shame because it is so beneficial (I would have included it in the section on wonder foods, if it were not for the pollution aspect). If you are not keen on chunks of liver, make a liver pâté (*see page 153*) – used as a spread or a dip it is delicious.

Conversely, do not serve liver too often to your child since it is so rich in vitamin A that you can overdo it. I would suggest once every second week from around the age of nine months is ideal.

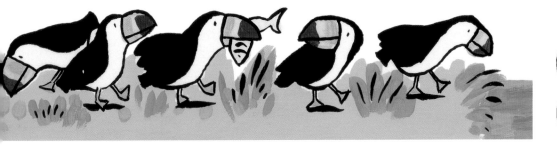

GOOD FOOD
ON A BUDGET

One of the criticisms levelled at 'healthy eating' is that you need to take out a mortgage to do it. This is simply not true and is really just an excuse for not making the effort. No doubt about it, it is an effort when compared to grabbing a supermarket-bought, ready-made meal from the freezer – but the results really are worth it, in terms of both your child's palate and long-term health.

The list of inexpensive foods that can appear on a health-conscious parent's shopping list are many:

Dried pulses, beans and grains are particularly nutritious, very filling and inexpensive. Compared to other protein sources like meat, they are ideal for a family on a budget, and meat can be a costly item to budget for. Choose from all the pulses and beans: red or brown lentils, chickpeas, black-eyed beans, kidney beans, butter beans, pinto beans and so on. The grains may be more familiar: brown rice, oats, wholewheat, rye, corn (maize) and barley; and some you may not have tried buckwheat, quinoa and millet.

Vegetables and fruit in season are the most economic bets. Root vegetables tend to be particularly inexpensive and are very filling and nutritious. Onions are cheap, can be used to jazz up all sorts of dishes and are one of the Wonder Foods (*see page 76*). At certain times of the year there are gluts of what is in season and produce is almost given away! If you have the time and energy you can blanch and freeze quantities of, for example, green beans, courgettes, broccoli, cauliflower and rhubarb, and fruits such as apples, plums and berries for pies or sauces.

Some fish are considerably less expensive than others: mackerel, herrings and sardines are extremely reasonable. Stock up by buying frozen fish – it keeps well, is nutritious, and cooks in 10–15 minutes when defrosted. And remember, oily fish are one of the Wonder Foods (*see page 76*).

Make good use of your freezer at all times of the year to freeze portions of stews. Cook them in larger batches than you need, and then freeze portion-sized servings for later use. They can be nutritious and use inexpensive ingredients such as beans and pulses. Also, it is actually quicker and easier to pull something out of the freezer than to shop for and cook convenience food options.

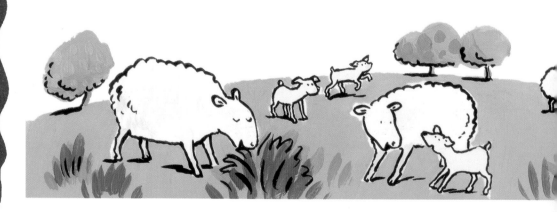

❧ ONE WEEK ON A BUDGET ❧

BREAKFASTS:
Oatmeal with raisins
Boiled egg and wholewheat 'soldiers'
Home-made muesli* with fresh seasonal fruit
Brown rice with grated apple, coconut flakes
     and soya milk
Wholegrain toast with nut butters
Quinoa-Millet Porridge*
Yoghurt with mashed banana & baby rice

LIGHT MEALS:
Thick Lentil and Tomato Soup with Rye Bread
Sardines on Wholewheat Toast
Home-made Hummus* with Vegetable Sticks
Coleslaw* and Oatcakes
Chunky Potato and Leek soup
Jacket Potato* and Filling
Baked Beans and Vegetarian Sausages
Pasta with Mushroom & Onion Sauce*

MAIN MEALS:
Barley stew* and chicken
Roasted Root Vegetables with Brown Rice
Vegetable Chilli*
Lemon Brussels Sprouts* with Quinoa*
     and Carrots
Coconut Fish Curry*
Bean & Garlic Stew*
Mediterranean Mackerel* and Vegetables

DESSERTS:
Baked apple stuffed with prunes
Banana soup*
Yoghurt and seasonal fruit
Indian Pudding*
Cinnamon wholewheat toast
Baked banana and yoghurt
Apple Cake*

See Recipe Index

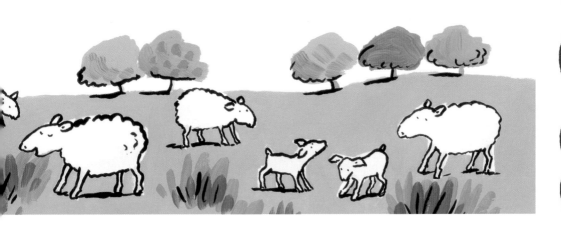

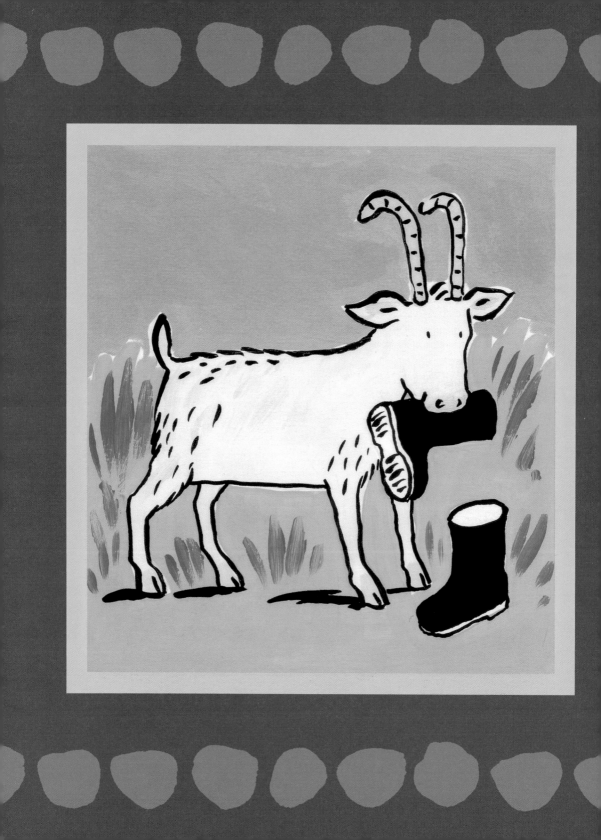

6

WHAT YOUR CHILD REALLY DOES NOT NEED

It would be lovely to write a book that concentrated solely on the positive value of eating from Nature's bounty. Sadly, as we live in the real world, this cannot be so. Our bodies and our chlidren's bodies, have to deal with excess levels of salt, sugar and hydrogenated fats so beloved of food manufacturers, toxic metals from pollution, and 3000 foreign chemicals that are added to our food supply.

WHY DO
CHILDREN LIKE SUGAR, SALT AND FATS?

The tug of war between parents and children about foods children would like to eat – crisps, sweets, cake, sausages – and what their parents would prefer them to eat – fruit, vegetables, 'proper meals' – will run and run. The food manufacturers know that we have a physiological predisposition to enjoy the taste sensations created by sugar, salt and fats and they play on it for all it is worth. What nature intended as a survival mechanism has been turned to advantage by food technologists.

The foods we are familiar with nowadays are completely different in their composition to those of only 100 years ago. The supermarkets offer a bewildering choice of attractively packaged products that make all sorts of impressive claims – reduced fat, low sugar, high fibre and so on.

As with many things, a little will probably not do that much harm, but food manufacturers know what makes us tick and go out of their way to produce products that have us, or our children, reaching for more. In particular, the food industry produces huge numbers of what are termed 'value-added foods' – they add sugar and fat, and the value (price) goes up! The fact is that sugar, salt and fat taste good. A major sector of the food industry is devoted to developing new ranges that accommodate our tastes for these substances – and the great advantage to the manufacturers is that these foods keep well on the shelves and use cheap ingredients. This makes it very profitable for them to put a lot of resources into this area. Many of these foods are deliberately designed to be appealing to children, while also appealing to parents because they are quick and convenient. They also will often make some carefully worded health claim such as 'low fat', 'sugar free' and so on.

Good, quick, healthy, snack-food options do exist – see the list on page 103.

SUGAR

There are two theories as to why we like sweet tastes. The first is that it is a survival mechanism inherited from our hunter-gatherer ancestors, since sweet fruit and berries are unlikely to be poisonous, whereas bitter ones might be. The other common theory is that we are designed to be fuelled by carbohydrates and so crave the sweetness of carbohydrate-loaded fruit and sweet root vegetables. The best way to satisfy sweet cravings, and in fact to regulate the whole mechanism involved in a taste for sweet foods, is to eat lots of delicious fruit.

Ingeniously, food manufacturers have reversed the benefit by refining sugars and so delivering a slow-working poison. Sugar really is the number one problem for any parent interested in their child's good health. Most parents know to keep juices and cordials to a minimum to preserve their child's teeth, but the impact of sugar on the whole body is adverse. To put it into perspective, sugar is a

❧ HIDDEN SUGAR ❧

COMMON PRODUCTS	SERVING SIZE	QUANTITY OF HIDDEN SUGAR
Fruit yoghurt	150 g/5 oz (1 small carton)	4 tsp
Baked beans	225 g/7½ oz (1 medium can)	2½ tsp
Canned sweetcorn	100 g/4 oz (⅓ can)	2 tsp
Tomato ketchup	10 g/⅓ oz (2 teaspoons)	½ tsp
Cornflakes	30 g/1¼ oz (3 tablespoons)	½ tsp
Canned tomato soup	200 g/7 oz (½ can)	1 tsp
Packet tomato soup	20 g/ ¾ oz (¼ packet)	2 tsp
Ice cream	50 g/2 oz (1 scoop)	2 tsp
Jam	15 g/ ½ oz (2 teaspoons)	2½ tsp
Low calorie drinks (specifying sugar on label)	40 ml/1½ fl oz (1 glass, diluted)	½ tsp

Hidden sugars are also called other things, so watch out for the following: glucose, maltose, sucrose, dextrose, lactose, galactose, fructose, hydrolysed starch, invert sugar, honey and concentrated fruit juice – to name but a few.

preservative. Why would you want to put a preservative into a young body?

Apart from damaging teeth there are other serious problems with sugar. You may have heard it said that sugar provides empty calories, but what does that mean? It means that sugar is devoid of any vitamins and minerals that would help the body to utilize it. For instance, we need a mineral, chromium, in order to metabolize sugar and yet not only does it not provide this mineral, it also causes a net loss of chromium from the body in the urine. So, over the years, people who consume sugar develop a deficiency of this nutrient. The calories that are provided have no vitamins or minerals to metabolize it, meaning that the body must draw on existing reserves.

This leads to another really serious problem with high sugar intake: impaired blood sugar control (see page 62). In some this can lead to adult diabetes and we are now seeing this form of diabetes in children for the first time. This is purely and simply a diet-related problem, which can be improved by keeping sugar to a minimum from a young age. Other serious complications that arise from excess sugar consumption include obesity, osteoporosis (since sugar increases calcium excretion from the body), suppressed immunity and cardiovascular disease.

The average person in the UK and USA consumes about 45.5 kg/100 lb of sugar a year; in France the figure is about 7 kg/15 lb, so cultural attitudes to food are obviously important. The sugar does not always come from adding spoonfuls of the stuff to food. It is more usually hidden in the foods we eat. The chart (*above*) provides a list of some of the hidden sugar in common products that children eat.

❧ THE TASTE OF HONEY ❧

Many people use honey, instead of sugar. However, while it does have some trace nutrients that may be useful, it is metabolized by the body in more or less the same way as sugar, and has the same impact on teeth. There is also a slight risk of botulism infection from honey and it therefore must be best avoided before the age of one year as babies do not have the right protective intestinal bacteria to fight it. For older children Manuka honey has useful antibiotic properties.

Sources of sweetness that are all right to use in moderation include finely chopped dried fruit, diluted freshly made fruit juices, a small amount of fructose and blackstrap molasses.

❧ ARTIFICIAL SWEETENERS ❧

Many products are sold as 'sugar free' or with 'reduced sugar', but to make up the sweetness they rely on artificial sweeteners. These are chemical compounds that have no place in a child's diet. They have to be processed by the body, stored, detoxified and eliminated. In excess quantities they can lead to metabolic imbalances.

Below are some of the most frequently used sweeteners to look out for:

Saccharine: Labelling on packages in the USA states 'Use of this product may be hazardous to your health. This product contains saccharine, which has been determined to cause cancer in laboratory animals.' Need I say more?

Aspartame: This is a di-peptide (two linked amino acids) which means that the manufacturers claim it is metabolized by the body. The only people cautioned against its use are those with PKU – for which all babies are tested at birth. However, its breakdown products are methanol, which can cause blindness in large quantities, and formaldehyde, a known carcinogen. These breakdown products occur after two or three months of storage or on application of heat. Some research is now showing a link with increased risk of brain tumours. The USDA recommend a maximum adult intake of methanol of 7.8 mg a day, and one can of diet soda will contain about twice that amount. Aspartame accounts for about 75% of the adverse food reactions reported to the US FDA (Food and Drug Administration).

Sorbitol: This is found in most diabetic products such as jams and sweets. It is an insoluble sugar end-product, crystals of which are found built up in the lens of the eye in those with cataracts. It is not certain that dietary sorbitol leads to this, but I would not want to take the risk with my child. In any event it is probably more sensible, for both diabetics and children, to curb a sweet tooth by changing habits rather than promoting it with sweeteners.

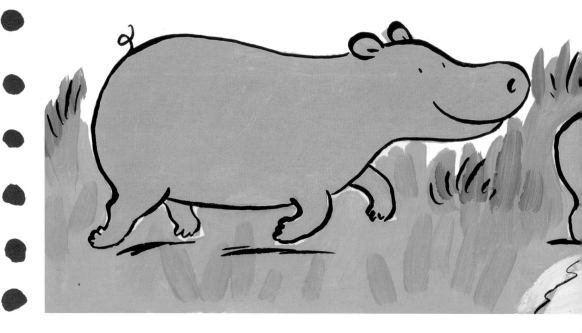

SALT

The salt question is quite a different one. Once upon a time, salt was so scarce that it was used as currency to pay the troops (hence the term 'sal-ary') and we do need sodium – our body is a saline medium. Our forebears lived on a fruit- and vegetable-rich diet, which gave them a lot of vital potassium and a small amount of the equally vital sodium. The sodium was in much lower quantity than the potassium – the ratio was about 4:1 potassium to sodium. Therefore, the probability is that our bodies evolved to retain selectively the scarce but necessary sodium by being reabsorbed by our kidneys, while the potassium was excreted since it was so plentiful. Nowadays, the reverse is true. We do not eat as much fruit and vegetables as our ancestors, but we sprinkle our food liberally via the salt cellar or buy manufactured foods that use salt in quantity. The modern diet has reversed the ratio to 4:1 sodium to potassium. This reversal has led to health problems like mineral imbalance, water retention and, more seriously, heart disease. For small children in particular, it is a problem since their kidneys do not cope well with a lot of added salt. The taste for salt can be satisfied with strong-tasting herbs and spices, and naturally salty foods such as seaweeds, fish roe and uneboshi dried plums – the organic sodium in these foods does not behave metabolically in the same way as the inorganic salt that we add to our food.

SALT FREE

Again, we have a taste for salt as a survival mechanism since we do actually need sodium, in small quantities and in the organic form found in plant life.

Salt consumption has been blown out of proportion in our food supply and consumption is at dangerously high levels. Children can get all the natural organic sodium they need from a fruit- and vegetable-rich diet.

Unfortunately the sins of the parent are often visited on the child, since we taste food destined for them and, finding it bland, will add salt – wrongly. There really is no need to add salt to food for children. Now is the time to experiment with herbs and spices. They have the advantage of being salt free; they develop your child's taste buds to accept

🐞 BEING PRACTICAL 🐞

It is not always practical to avoid some salty foods that lend interest to recipies, such as olives, soya sauce and anchovies. Used in moderation they are fine.

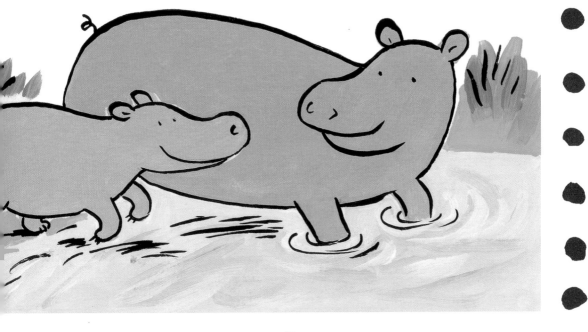

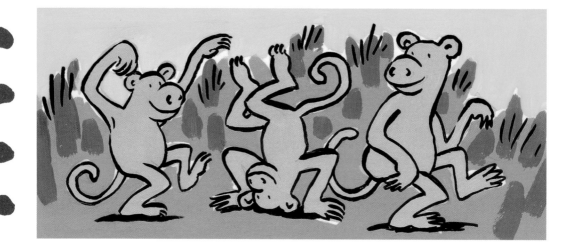

❦ CAFFEINE ❦

One of the most disturbing sights I think I have ever seen is an 18-month-old child being wheeled in his pram suckling on a bottle filled with a cola drink.

Cola contains caffeine which is addictive and, as far as I am concerned, should be a controlled substance for anyone under the age of 16. It acts as a potent central nervous system stimulator and can cause restlessness, nervousness and insomnia. The colossal sales of cola drinks testify to their attractive qualities, but colas, chocolate drinks and popular glucose drinks – all with high caffeine and sugar or artificial sweetener contents – should be avoided. No child needs them.

a wide variety of foods, and many of the herbs and spices have protective and therapeutic qualities. Herbs and spices that have strong flavours and are ideal substitutes for salt include coriander leaves, tarragon, basil, mint, cumin, paprika, chives and seaweed flakes. You can also get sodium- and monosodium glutamate-free bouillon cubes from good health food shops.

FAT

Research is now showing that we may be programmed to eat fat, also as a survival mechanism, in our quest for the essential fats which are vital in our diet. The research suggests that if this is not satisfied with essential fats, and we use the non-essential saturated fats as alternatives, the need for them is really never met. So we just carry on eating fats. Eat enough of the essential fats and the natural balancing act of taste versus satiety should eventually be restored. Satisfy your child's fat requirements with extra-virgin olive oil, fresh ground seeds, cold-pressed vegetable oils and oily fish.

FEARSOME FATS

All fats are not equal. The fats to keep to a minimum in the case of a small child are those that interfere with the good fats, which are needed for brain and nervous tissue development, cell membrane structure and hormone production. The greatest culprits are hydrogenated fats found in margarines and processed foods. The truth is that the beneficial, health-giving oils have such a short shelf-life – they must be fresh in order to work – that they are no friend of food manufacturers. The food industry likes foods that are cheap and have a long shelf life, and so use hydrogenated fats in preference to others. Oil that is heated will also interfere with the positive benefits of the good oils. Olive oil is less susceptible to damage but do not let it smoke. For cooking it is therefore important to use a little butter or olive oil . Oils are best kept refrigerated to prevent oxidation damage. It is not appropriate for a child to have a low-fat diet – as is the trend with many adults. This is because children have small stomachs in relation to their energy needs and need the calories gained from useful fats. The chart opposite lists various fat and oil sources and their best uses.

❦ SOURCES AND USES OF FATS AND OILS ❦

FAT	TYPE	USES
Butter		Cooking
Margarine (most brands)	Hydrogenated	Do not use
Margarine (e.g. Granose)	Emulsified/non-hydrogenated	Spreading
Olive oil	Extra-virgin, cold pressed	Cooking or salads/sauces
Sunflower oil	Cold pressed; do not heat; refrigerate	Salads or add to cooled dishes for flavour
Safflower oil	Cold pressed; do not heat; refrigerate	Salads or add to cooled dishes for flavour
Walnut, almond, hazelnut and other nut oils	Cold pressed; do not heat; refrigerate	Salads or add to cooled dishes for flavour
Flax oil	Cold pressed; do not heat; refrigerate	Salads or add to cooled dishes
Peanut (groundnut) oil		May contain toxins (*see page 65*) and implicated in heart disease; do not use
Corn oil		Low oil content in corn means extraction uses very high temperatures and toxic solvents; do not use
Sesame oil		Contains sesamol, which makes it very stable; stir-fries
Nuts and seeds	Fresh, unroasted; refrigerate	Snacks
Tahini		As a spread
Nut and seed butters	Almond, cashew, sunflower seed; refrigerate	As spreads
Peanut butter	Use organic, sugar- and salt-free brands	Use sparingly (*see page 65*)

LABELS
AND HOW TO READ THEM

This, believe it or not, is a well-known brand of children's dessert – banana flavour! I could not find the banana – and very little else that even remotely resembles food with any nutrient value.

Three thousand different chemicals are added to our food and, on average, each of us consumes 6.5 kg/14 lb of chemicals a year! There is nothing for it but to be a detective if you want to protect your child from the worst of these. Many people feel that they cannot spend their whole time in the supermarket reading labels, but a judicious look at the key ingredients will say a lot, and after you have done the groundwork you learn to avoid some brands and to go for others.

Here are the main pointers to look out for:

Ingredient order: Labels will always list ingredients in order of quantity. So if the bolognaise sauce you are buying says: 'tomato, starch, onion, meat, herbs…' you know that the meat content is virtually the lowest by weight – probably a good thing, but not necessarily what you think you are buying.

Hidden sugar: This ingredient is often disguised by calling it anything but sugar. The basic rule is that any word that ends in '-ose' or '-ol' is a sugar: maltose, glucose, lactose, galactose, sucrose, fructose and sorbitol (*see page 87*). Anything that says syrup is also a sugar, such as corn syrup.

Maltodextrin is a partially broken-down carbohydrate, halfway between a starch and a sugar. When fully hydrolysed it is used for the gum on the back of stamps and envelopes; partially hydrolysed it finds its way into many foods, including baby foods. Maltodextrin is a cheap, bulking agent. It has no food value, and in the final analysis is broken down into sugar. This does not help with keeping a taste for sweet foods at bay or with maintaining blood sugar balance.

Nitrites: All cured foods and some smoked foods, especially sausages, ham and bacon, will contain nitrites, which are preservatives. Nitrites convert to nitrosamines in the stomach, which are suspected of being cancer-producing chemicals. Preservatives are used to inhibit the development of mould, as mould can have very bad consequences for children. If you elect to give your children packaged foods, preservatives are something that you and they will have to put up with. However no preservatives are actually good for health, so the message here is to keep packaged foods to a minimum.

Emulsifiers: These are used principally to increase the water content of, for instance, meat, in order to increase profit margins for the food manufacturers. The emulsifier lecithin, which appears naturally in foods, is fine and is used to bind sauces. However, since most lecithin comes from soya, you should avoid this if your child is sensitive to soya products.

Antioxidants: These are necessary to stop foods from becoming rancid. They are present in nature and are an important part of our diet. Ascorbates (vitamin C) and tocopherol (vitamin E) are the good antioxidants that are used. However, ingeniously, the food-processing industry has managed to come up with a few other antioxidants that are problematic – these include BHA, BHT and gallates which may be carcinogenic.

Food colouring: This is simply not necessary. It is included to make food more marketable and appealing – and for no other reason. A couple – carotene (vitamin A) and riboflavin (vitamin B2) – are all right, others are not. I suggest you avoid the rest, on behalf of your child.

MSG: This is short for monosodium glutamate (E621), a relative of salt and is used as a flavour enhancer. Many people are sensitive to MSG and a whole syndrome has been described called 'Chinese Restaurant Syndrome'. Thankfully, it is no longer used in baby foods, but it still appears in many other packaged foods. Hydrolysed vegetable protein (HVP) is an additive that includes MSG and should therefore be kept to a minimum, or preferably avoided for small children.

FILLERS, PRESERVATIVES & ADDITIVES

Read any food product label and you are likely to see a list of unfathomable names.

Fillers add bulk (starch, modified starch and maltodextrine) and are the way in which food manufacturers keep the costs down. It is usually the case that you pay for what you get. If a packaged food is cheap, there is usually a reason.

Preservatives keep food from decomposing too soon. Sugar and salt are ancient preservatives, but now there is a chemical army of preservatives, including sorbates, benzoates and carbon dioxide, to mention a few unsavoury names.

Additives are mostly artificial flavourings and colourings. Some are harmful and some are not – frankly it is difficult for anyone without a degree in food chemistry to differentiate easily between them. Some 'E-numbers', for instance, are quite innocuous additives like vitamin C and E used to reduce oxidation of food. Some are quite harmful, however (see the chart opposite), and have been linked to specific childhood problems. For example, tartrazine, a yellow colouring, is implicated in hyperactivity and asthma.

It is interesting to note that in some countries E-number regulations are tighter than in others. E104, a yellow colouring commonly used in sweets and desserts, is banned in Norway, the USA, Australia and Japan. E110, another yellow colouring used in cordials and sweets, is banned in Norway and Finland. E124, a red colouring used in sweets, is banned in Norway and the USA because of the health risk for asthmatics.

I would suggest that you buy foods with the good E-numbers on the first list in the chart, avoid foods with the bad ones on the second list and, if possible, cut back as much as you can on the hundreds I have not listed because they have not definitively been shown to be either benevolent or overtly bad.

There are some good publications available that give all the information on E-numbers and additives, which are listed on page 185.

❧ E-NUMBERS ❧

In brief, the only E-numbers that are good for you and your child, or are necessary, are as follows:

Colourings
E101 Riboflavin, E160 Carotene

Preservatives
E200-E290 Necessary for food safety; not harmful, but not good either

Antioxidants
E300-E304 Ascorbates
E306-E309 Tocopherols

Emulsifiers, stabilizers and others
E322 Lecithin, E375 Nicotinic acid, E440 Pectin

The ones that are actually bad for you and your child are:

Colourings
E102, E104-142, E150, E151-E155, E173, E174

Preservatives
E200-E203, E210-E219, E220-E227, E230-E249, E250-E252, E262, E281-E283, E290

Antioxidants
E310-312, E320-321

Emulsifiers, stabilizers and others
E385, E407, E513, E525, E535, E541, E621, E631, E635, E905, E924, E925

PROTECTION
FROM POLLUTION

We now live in an environment that is completely different to the one in which we evolved. Our environment and food now deliver a huge range of substances that, in large quantities, can cause havoc – especially in the young, developing child. The average person in the UK breathes in 1 g of what are called 'heavy metals' a year. Imagine a 1 g weight on an old-fashioned weighing machine! Heavy metals are also antinutrients, which means that they block the positive use of nutrients from our food.

Keeping exposure to a minimum is one of the best things that you can do for your child, and here are some of the protective measures you can take against the worst offenders.

LEAD
This is one of the worst substances for the developing child, since it is a known neurotoxin – in other words it poisons nervous tissue. This is the reason that leaded paint was banned for use on toys. Current Government figures show that one in ten children have high blood lead levels sufficient to impair IQ. The situation has improved since the use of leaded petrol has been dramatically reduced. However, there is still quite a lot of air-borne lead pollution in our environment. Another major source is the lead pipework in old houses, so it is a good idea to check that your water supply is not delivered through lead pipes. Lead, a poison, and zinc, a nutrient, are directly antagonistic to each other. This means that, if a child has good zinc levels, lead absorption is kept to a minimum.

CADMIUM
Most parents are on guard against exposing their children to cigarette smoke these days, especially now that definite links have been made with cot deaths. But, if you need another reason to avoid tobacco, cigarettes are one of the chief sources of cadmium, which is a toxic metal.

MERCURY
We all know about the mad hatter in Alice in Wonderland (in the old days, hatters commonly went insane because mercury was used in the hat-making process). Our main exposure to mercury comes from pesticides and amalgam tooth fillings. Children under the age of two are unlikely to have any fillings but it is an important decision whether or not to allow your children to have amalgam fillings, and one you should discuss with your dentist carefully. There is an ongoing debate about this issue at the moment, and it is interesting that some European countries have banned its use already, or have plans to do so in the next few years. The alternative option is to have composite fillings.

ALUMINIUM
Important sources of contamination are aluminium foil, antiperspirants, antacid medication and aluminium cooking vessels, especially when used with acidic foods such as lemon, tomatoes or rhubarb that leach the metal. A link between aluminium and Alzheimer's disease is always under review. It is unclear at the moment if the levels of aluminium in the brain of sufferers is a cause or an effect.

COPPER
This is actually an essential nutrient but, in excess, it acts as an antinutrient. The main exposure for children comes from copper water pipes, especially when newly installed and before they have had a chance to 'fur up'. If your house does have new copper pipes you may want to consider using a water filter or bottled water.

❧ STEPS TO AVOID EXPOSURE ❧

The following are steps you can take to ensure you keep your child's exposure to pollutants to a minimum:

❧ Keep packaged foods to a minimum.

❧ Buy organic foods if you can.

❧ If you do not buy organic, wash all fruit and vegetables. A capful of vinegar in a bowl of water helps to break down the waxy residue that is on most fruit. Remove the outer leaves of vegetables.

❧ Avoid fresh foods that are subject to roadside pollution, such as from market stalls on busy roads.

❧ Avoid copper or aluminium cookware and aluminium food wrapping. Use stainless steel or ceramic cookware and storage containers.

❧ Do not drink or cook with water processed through a water softener as soft water dissolves lead more readily (this is not related to salts used in water softeners). If you are drinking or cooking with tap water ensure you are using water that comes directly from the mains supply.

❧ Use a water filter or, if possible, drink distilled or mineral water.

❧ Keep the use of over-the-counter medication to a minimum – antacids, for example, contain aluminium.

❧ Make sure that small children do not pick at, or chew on, paintwork.

❧ Avoid soft plastic food wrapping (clingfilm). Certainly do not use it to wrap food closely. It leaches a damaging oestrogenic compound called nonylphenol into fats in food.

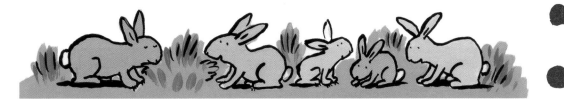

❧ NUTRIENTS THAT DETOXIFY ❧

Some nutrients and foods are very good at getting rid of heavy metals:

Calcium and phosphorous are antagonistic to lead. Nuts, seeds and green leafy vegetables are rich in these minerals. Calcium is also antagonistic to cadmium and aluminium.

Vitamin C conducts lead, cadmium and arsenic out of the body. Fruit that are richest in vitamin C are citrus fruit, kiwi fruit, blackcurrants and strawberries. Vitamin C-rich vegetables include cabbage, bean sprouts, peppers, potatoes and sweet potatoes.

Zinc is an antagonist of lead and cadmium. Good sources include egg yolks, sardines, chicken, almonds, cucumber, buckwheat, peas and liver.

Magnesium is good for detoxifying aluminium. Food sources are all green leafy vegetables, as well as garlic, onions, tomatoes, prunes, aubergines, apricots, sweetcorn and potatoes with their skins .

Sulphur amino acids help protect against lead, cadmium and mercury. They are found in eggs, onions and garlic.

Pectin helps to get rid of lead and can be found in apples, bananas, citrus fruit and carrots.

Alginic acid comes from seaweed and is a very potent lead detoxifier. Dried seaweed flakes are available from good health food shops and can be used as a savoury seasoning on all sorts of dishes.

ALLERGIES
& FOOD SENSITIVITIES

When talking about food, the term 'allergy' is generally used to describe any adverse reaction. Strictly speaking, this is not quite accurate. An allergy is a very specific reaction involving an immediate immune response to a food. This immune response is technically described as an IgE, or Type I, allergy and can be very nasty – even fatal – for the sufferer.

A serious immune reaction does not usually become apparent at the first exposure to the food, or other trigger. This is the time when the immune response is being 'programmed' by the body. The major response is more likely to happen on the second or subsequent exposures and can involve an extreme reaction by the body.

Avoiding exposure in the early years can reduce the risk of developing such allergies. You cannot, however, always be certain that your child is not being exposed. Therefore, in view of the potential danger of such a reaction, it may be best to find out if your child is at risk in controlled circumstances. Many parents will avoid foods like peanuts, but they may be unaware of their child being exposed at other times. For instance, peanuts are used in many products and are not always described on the package as 'peanuts' – they may be called groundnuts or the ingredients may list groundnut oil. It could even be that there are no peanuts in the product but the manufacturing machinery has been used for another product that uses peanuts, and some residue is left behind. A serious allergy can be so sensitive that this residue will be picked up.

My view is that, with the high-risk foods, I would rather expose my child at a time when we are close to a doctor's office and during opening hours – remembering that it is the second exposure that is most likely to trigger the reaction. If there is a serious reaction you can get your child to the doctor's office for treatment immediately.

If it is the case that your child has this type of allergy he will probably have that immune reaction for life. The only answer is to avoid the food. In some cases the child can be referred by the doctor to a specialist to be desensitized.

Peanuts are highest on the list of foods that may trigger a serious allergy and, if being super-cautious, are probably best left until the age of five years. They are a concentrated source of lectins, which are protein molecules that bind to human cells. This may be why they can cause such a serious reaction. If your child tends towards allergy, or comes from a family that does, then it may be wise to protect him from this small risk. Be aware also that peanut or groundnut oil can provoke the same reaction and, because it is found in so many products including nappy creams, this may be the reason why the number of children that are becoming sensitized is on the increase. Parents who are concerned about the small risk of this and other life-threatening allergies should seek guidance from their doctor or one of the allergy associations listed on page 184.

The Meal-Planners in this book have been grouped by age in order to help you to introduce high-risk foods in sequence.

❧ WHEEZERS & SNEEZERS ❧

There can be a familial tendency to allergy reactions such as hay fever, eczema, asthma, psoriasis, migraines and colitus. This trait is called 'atopy' and sufferers are described as coming from 'atopic' families. Therefore, if there is such a history in your family, including grandparents and aunts and uncles, then it is wise to take even more care with the introduction of foods that can provoke allergy or sensitivity. This is because they can act as triggers or can destabilize metabolism sufficiently to induce these allergic symptoms.

FOOD SENSITIVITIES AND INTOLERANCES

A food sensitivity is quite a different situation but is, confusingly – and some would say incorrectly, sometimes referred to as an allergy. The effect may involve an immune IgG, or delayed Type II, reaction – as opposed to the instant immune reaction described above. There may not even be an immune component to the reaction at all if it is an intolerance. Dietarily speaking, we can only be allergic to proteins, so there may also be intolerances as is the case with lactose (milk sugar) intolerance.

Whatever the type of reaction, food sensitivities and intolerances work in a more subtle way than classic allergies, undermining health and disrupting normal functioning. In children this type of reaction can contribute to eczema, asthma, hay fever, colic, mouth ulcers, bloating, diarrhoea, constipation, rashes, psoriasis, stomach pains, excess wind and behavioural problems.

A small child's digestive tract is more permeable than an adult's, meaning that there is a potential for larger, not fully digested molecules to cross the barrier. Some foods tend to cause more harm than others in this way.

If care is taken about restricting exposure to the possible problem foods at an early stage, the foods can usually be introduced at a later stage without harm, as long as they are not eaten to excess.

❦ PROBLEM FOODS ❦

The most common foods to cause problems with intolerance or sensitivity are:

❦ Wheat – it could be the wheat itself or it could be the gluten in the wheat (or more correctly the protein, gliadin, found in the gluten).

❦ Dairy products – it could be the lactose (milk sugar) or the milk proteins that cause the problems.

❦ Other grains, including oats, barley and rye which also contain gluten.

❦ Soya products.

❦ Citrus fruit, especially oranges.

❦ Corn and other low-gluten grains such as rice.

❦ Eggs – especially the whites. Well-cooked yolks can be introduced first and, if tolerated, you can then move on to cooked whites.

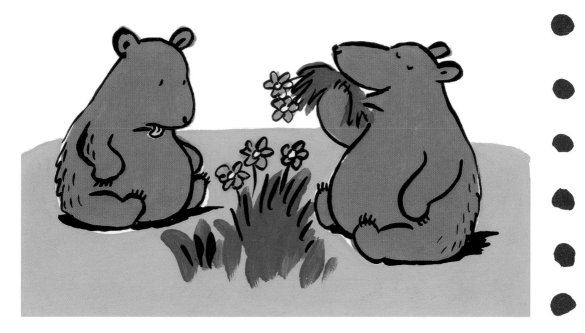

❦ IN-SEQUENCE PROGRAMME ❦

Below is the ideal order in which to introduce foods, one stage at a time.

AGE 4-8 MONTHS:

1 Vegetables (except the deadly nightshade group – see 9 right)
2 Fruit (except citrus)
3 Pulses and beans
4 Rice, buckwheat, quinoa and millet
5 Poultry, meat and fish*
6 Egg yolks

AGE 9-14 MONTHS:

7 Oats, barley, corn and rye
8 Live yoghurt

9 Deadly nightshade family (potatoes, tomatoes, aubergines, peppers)
10 Whole eggs*
11 Soya products*
12 Shellfish*

AGE 15-24 MONTHS:

13 Oranges
14 Wheat
15 Dairy products
16 Seeds* and nuts* (not peanuts)

AGE 5 YEARS:

17 Peanuts*

*The foods marked with an asterisk are those most commonly associated with the classical Type I food allergy (as opposed to food intolerance or sensitivity). Do remember that the protein component of any food can provoke this sort of reaction. I have erred on the side of caution and chosen to put these foods in at stages when most children can tolerate them. If you are happy to take the risk, you may want to introduce them a little earlier as they are all good nutritious foods. For example, I chose to give my son finely ground sunflower seeds, pumpkin seeds and fresh nuts from the age of around eight months as I believed the risk was small, but the nutritional benefits were many. On the other hand, I was very strict with grains and dairy because of the far greater risk of sensitivity becoming a problem.

INTRODUCING FOODS IN SEQUENCE

The worrying thing about a list like the one above is that these are the foods that are most commonly given to a small child – a bottle of milk and a rusk, orange juice and scrambled eggs. At this point most parents begin to panic and wonder what they can give their children.

The object of the exercise is to introduce foods in the order in which they are likely to do the least damage to the digestive tract, and to avoid setting up sensitivities, or allergies, especially if you suspect that your child might be prone to them. The ultimate objective is that your child should enjoy a fully varied diet in which all, or at least most, foods can be enjoyed in moderation.

If, after following such a programme, you find that your child is not the type to have food sensitivities, rejoice and pat yourself on the back, because you will have discovered a lot of different types of foods for him to eat without falling into the nutritional pitfall of following a diet based on too restricted a list of ingredients.

TAKE NOTES

Keep a food diary to note any new foods you introduce and any adverse reactions that your child experiences. If you suspect a food, withdraw it and reintroduce it a couple of weeks later. If you notice a pattern then avoid that food for several months before testing it again. Obviously do not reintroduce

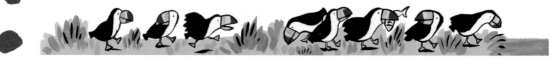

foods to which your child has had a severe or dangerous reaction.

You may also find that your child begins to have a reaction to a food that he has been eating for a while. This is often because it has been eaten too frequently and a threshold of reaction has been reached. In this instance I would suspect an IgG reaction. The IgG antibody has a 'short-term memory', which can be fooled into not responding. I suggest you avoid giving him the food totally for about eight weeks, not even the tiniest bit – read product labels for hidden traces. After that you may find that a four- or five-day rotation of the food avoids the problem of 'reprogramming' and you can avoid symptoms in your child. In other words, keep that food for 'high days and holidays' only.

❧ WHEAT AND DAIRY ALTERNATIVES ❧

By far the worst culprits for food sensitivities are wheat and dairy food. If you suspect this is the case with your child then here are the possible alternatives:

WHEAT ALTERNATIVES:

Oats	porridge, oatcakes, oat muesli
Rye	rye crispbreads, pumpernickel, flat dark German rye bread
Rice	brown rice, rice cakes, pasta, as a breakfast dish with coconut and chopped dried fruit
Corn	tortillas, nachos, popcorn, pasta, pastry, baked goods
Barley	made like rice, pasta
Buckwheat	blinis, flour, noodles, pasta (not wheat, despite the name)
Quinoa	made like rice, cereal
Millet	cereal, porridge
Spelt flour/bread	this is actually wheat, but an ancient strain of the grain which some can tolerate
Bulgar wheat	also wheat, but a different sort that some can tolerate
Chickpea flour	gram flour
Lentil flour	poppadums
Almonds	ground, useful for cereals and baking
Muesli	made with a variety of grains, seeds, nuts and chopped dried fruit
Sauce thickening	corn, barley, gram, rice or potato flours
Potatoes and rice dishes	starchy foods that substitute for pasta dishes

DAIRY ALTERNATIVES:

Soya milk	best for making porridge and on cereals (choose calcium-enriched)
Rice milk	a refreshing drink and good on cereals (choose calcium-enriched)
Oat milk	good for baking (choose calcium-enriched)
Almond milk	use as an alternative to cream
Coconut milk	a good alternative to cream, and excellent in sauces; very rich so dilute 50/50, or to taste
Soya yoghurt and cheese	live yoghurts available
Butter	100% fat so usually tolerated by those with a dairy allergy
Whey milk	for milk shakes; usually tolerated by those with dairy allergy as reaction is usually to the casein protein and not the whey component

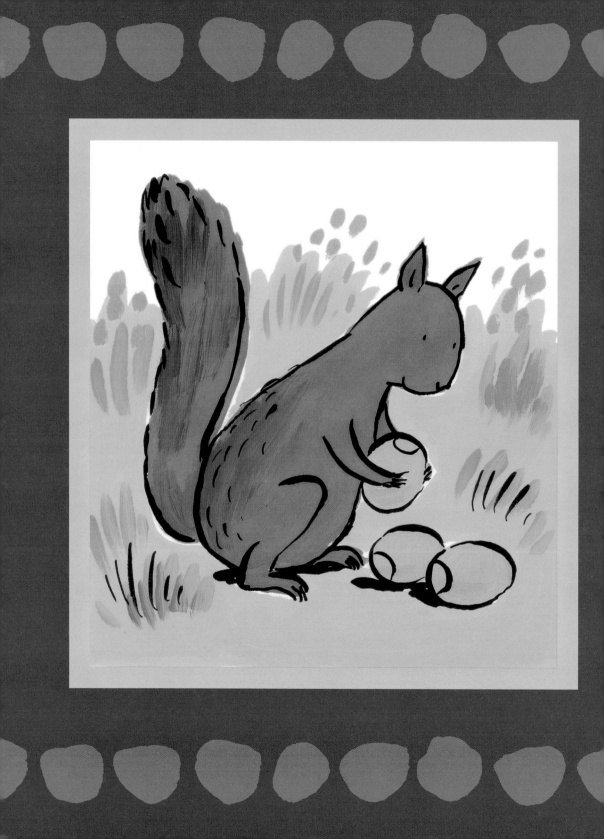

7

THE EASY OPTIONS

B eing interested in health and healthy eating does not mean that you do not have the same needs as any other time-pressed parent. Supermarkets and health food shops are stocked with snacks that make all sorts of reassuring health statements. Unfortunately, they tend not to live up to their claims, and are full of hydrogenated fats and preservatives. In particular, we tend to be lulled by the words 'health food shop' into believing that everything they stock is healthy. It is not necessarily so – you need to be selective. Always read the list of ingredients!

FAST FOOD
NOT JUNK FOOD

The era of fast food is upon us. But fast is not necessarily bad – it just helps to be able to differentiate between them. A can of sardines, some wholemeal pasta shells, a baked potato, frozen peas and sweetcorn or a tub of mackerel pâté are all fast – and nourishing. With the correct information it is quite easy to make good choices when in a rush. Equally fast, and to be viewed with suspicion, are shaped re-textured chicken nuggets, high-street hamburgers, processed cheese slices and the majority of sausages.

BABY FOODS

Jars of baby food are a great temptation. Even the most health-conscious parents probably think about using some of the foods that are on offer. However, the majority of baby food in jars or packets are fairly unsatisfactory. At least they are no longer full of salt or colouring but they are frequently thickened with fillers that have no nutritious value at all and provide only empty calories, and many of them contain sugar in one form or another.

A recent report by the Food Commission found that the majority of baby foods were being bulked out with low-nutrient starches. The report showed that 54% contained unnecessary, non-milk sugars (19% of the foods containing sugars were savoury products); 60% contained low-nutrient fillers such as maltodextrin and modified cornflour; and 17% of baby foods for those under four months old contained gluten, despite the fact that the UK government has recommended that foods for babies under six months should be gluten free.

It is always worth reading the list of contents since you may not be buying what you think you are. For example, one baby food product from a major company is called 'Cheese, spinach and potato bake', implying that cheese is a main constituent – probably playing on most parents' concern that their child receives sufficient calcium. Read the contents list and you will find that cheese actually comes 11th on the ingredients list and it turns out that there is more maltodextrin, a low-nutrient filler, in the product than there is cheese.

Due to growing consumer demand some product lines are now offering organic baby foods, including some of the chain store brands. It is worth trying them as new formulations come on to the market all the time. Brands include Organix, Hipp, Boots Mothers' Recipe and Cow and Gate Organic Choice.

The only range I have found that gives me everything I am looking for in a prepared baby food is the Organix range. The product actually tastes good – I always urge parents to taste from the jar they are giving their child to see if this is the taste they want their child to develop. The Organix products are organic, mostly avoid foods on the sensitivity list, and use no fillers or sugars. They are available from quite a few major supermarkets, and if you cannot find them, their address is on page 184. Pleasingly, other brands are beginning to follow their lead. Another option is the American brand, Beech-Nut, available in some shops. It is not organic, but they use simple ingredients, in stages, using no fillers, sugars or potential allergens.

My overall view on jars of baby food is that the best-quality ones are fine as an occasional standby, but I do not suggest that they are used as a substitute for 'real food' too often. One way to cheat a little, and to keep a moderately clear conscience, is to keep some frozen cubes of cooked red lentils or brown rice in the freezer (*see Recipe Index*) and mix them in with the jar of baby food to increase the nutrient value. You can also grate a little carrot, cucumber or apple into the food to give it a fresh food boost.

If you do use prepared foods keep them to a minimum. Freshly prepared food will educate your child's palate to enjoy real food and you can control the ingredients.

❦ HEALTHY SNACKS ❦

If the only change you make to your family's eating habits is to ensure that they have healthy snack options instead of the standard choices, you would be doing so much good – and they are easier than you may think. With a little forethought it is quite simple to have a number of healthy standbys available for a quick snack – to grab before going out or to form the basis of a light meal with some shredded vegetables and quick dip pots, like guacamole or salsa. Here are a few suggestions:

❦ I find that offering a piece of fruit is almost always well received.

❦ Crudités – cucumber, red and yellow peppers, carrots and mushrooms are delicious with a dip or just on their own.

❦ Flavoured mini rice crackers and mini poppadums are available from health food shops and are a good alternative to crisps.

❦ Muffins, home-made and sugar free, can be made in bulk and frozen. Grab a few when you are going out to provide sustenance for hungry little (or big) people.

❦ An easy option is to put a bowl of cereals in front of your little one. Why not? Grains are nutritious and can sustain an appetite into the next meal. Sugar-free cereals are really the only option in my view and might include porridge, sugar-free cornflakes or Kashi multi-grain (the last two are available from health food shops). Add a little chopped fruit and some milk – preferably soya, rice or oat milk – and you have a quick, filling snack.

❦ Oatcakes and mini rice cakes can be bought from most supermarkets. They can be spread with 100% fruit spread, sunflower seed spread, nut butters, tahini, hummus, salsa or a little cottage cheese.

❦ Popcorn can be made in minutes – sprinkle with cinnamon for added flavour.

❦ Raisins and dried fruit are a great standby, although preferably not too often since they are very sweet. I suggest buying the unsulphured variety and you can try apple rings, apricots, prunes, pineapple rings and others.

❦ Plain yoghurt jazzed up with some cut-up fresh fruit is a good quick snack.

❦ Low-salt corn chips, on occasion, are good with guacamole, salsa, yoghurt and cucumber dip or refried beans.

❦ Wholegrain breadsticks are a good standby to munch on or to use for dips.

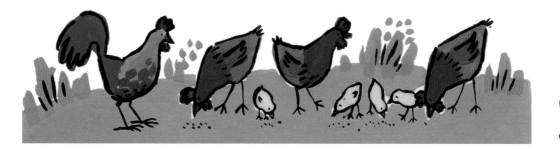

ON THE MOVE,
IN A RUSH...

Fast meals, that need almost no preparation and can be put into a box for a meal-on-the-move, can be perfectly good nutritionally speaking. Just because they are quick does not mean they are bad.

Suggestions could include the following:

♥ Hummus, home-made or shop bought, can be eaten from a spoon, and does not have to be spread on bread. It is made from puréed chickpeas and sesame paste, and so is high in minerals and fibre, making it a satisfying and healthy fast food.

♥ Sardines in tomato sauce mashed up on wholemeal toast, provides a good dose of essential fats and the antioxidant lycopene along with some fibre and B-vitamins in the toast.

♥ The much maligned and humble baked bean is a sound source of protein, fibre and minerals – although I would use the reduced sugar and salt organic brands.

♥ Frozen peas have been advertised as VIPs (very important peas!) with justification. They contribute around 9 g of fibre per half cup and are also an important source of zinc. Mixed with frozen sweetcorn they make a colourful and nutritious, almost instant, vegetable.

♥ Salmon mayonnaise is a valuable way of getting calcium into your child. Perhaps reduce the amount of mayonnaise and add some vinaigrette or yoghurt for a healthier option.

♥ Omelettes, cold and cut into chunks, Spanish style, make good finger food. Flavours to try are: herb, mushroom (see Recipe Index), tomato, salmon, onion or potato or any mixture of these.

♥ Ready-made falafels, or packets of falafel mix, are delicious and nutritionally sound. Bake the ready-made ones or lightly fry the ones you make up in olive oil. Traditionally, they are served with a 'salata' made from finely diced tomato, cucumber and onion, stirred through with some tahini and

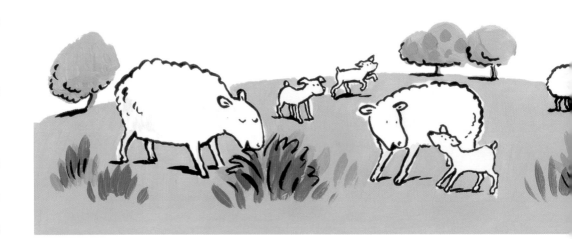

lemon juice – a very refreshing accompaniment that can be made in five minutes. If you want you can fit all this into a wholemeal pitta bread pocket, although it may be a bit messy for a little one – try serving with pitta bread sliced into fingers instead.

Vegetarian nuggets and sausages can be bought from the freezer section of most supermarkets and health food stores. They are not ideal, but they are not terrible either. At least they offer fibre, protein and minerals – not great as staples but fine for standbys.

What I call the 'quickie counter' in most supermarkets offers a range of reasonably healthy dips and salads. Select from hummus, guacamole, salsa dip, bean dip, coleslaw, three-bean salad and olives. They make a good easy mezze with vegetables and crackers to dip in them. This can be a bit messy with younger children, but they will enjoy the different shapes and textures and it is quick, fun and tasty.

Fresh soups in milk carton-type containers can be found in most large supermarkets. They use fresh ingredients, the packaging process retains most of the nutrients, and they also freeze well to use as standbys. Most of them are wheat free and many are also dairy free. You could, of course, have your own home-made soups on standby in the freezer.

Pasta is the regular standby that is trotted out time and again. I would recommend wholewheat pasta, and then only in moderation, since it is so easy to establish a sensitivity to wheat that can plague your child in later years. I strongly suggest you try pasta made from other grains in order to reduce the potential of this problem. Corn, millet, buckwheat and rice pasta are available from health food shops. The best options for children are the pasta shapes, shells or twists, and you can often find them in different colours – the colourings are natural. Flavour them with a sauce you keep in the freezer for a quick meal (*see Recipe Index*) – my son's favourite is tomato, anchovy and olive.

Brown rice is an excellent staple since it is filling, nutritious and a good base for many dishes, both savoury and sweet. It is a bore to cook though as it takes around 40 minutes, which is particularly irritating for small quantities. However, I do have a solution. It freezes very well. Freeze it in portion sizes and, after defrosting, heat it thoroughly and it is ready to serve. Alternatively you could use cous-cous which cooks in five minutes. See the Recipe Index for rice dish ideas.

Jacket potatoes with fillings of all descriptions are filling and quick. As long as the skin is eaten, they are good sources of complex carbohydrates, folic acid, vitamin C and B-vitamins. For a list of delicious suggested fillings see page 151.

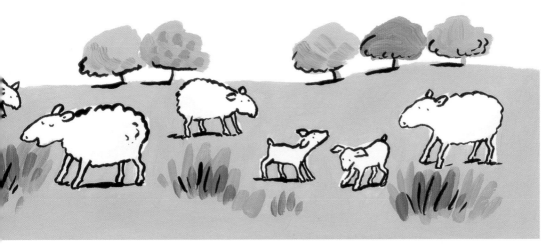

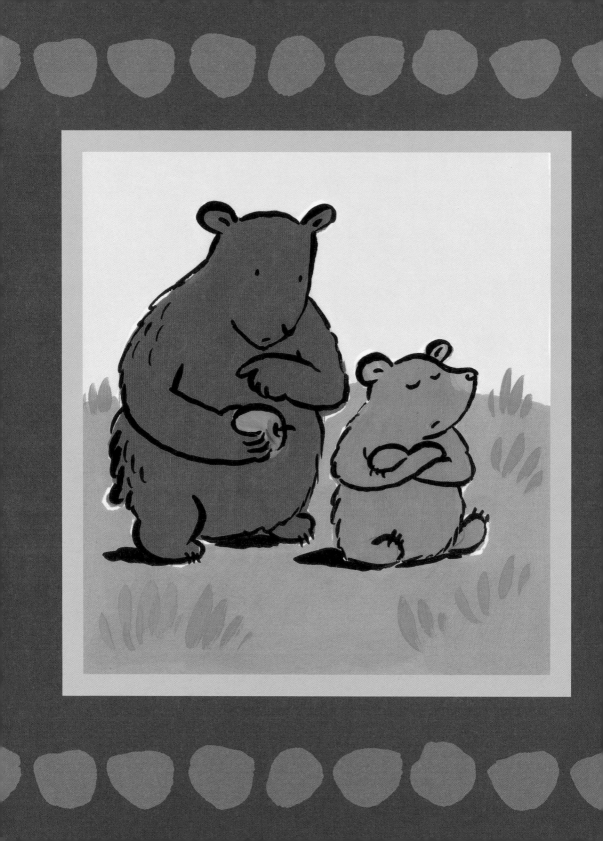

8

FOOD WARS

So many of our senses play a part in the consumption of food – the taste of food, the smell of food, the look and the texture of food. Meal times can be the most pleasurable and entertaining of social occasions and they reconfirm, at every sitting, the closeness of the family unit.

This may all sound somewhat idealistic to harassed parents who are worried that their child is not eating enough of the right foods, at the right time, in the right circumstances. Meal times are often the scene of the worst pitched battles in the home, although they do not have to be…

HAPPY
MEAL TIMES

Eating is not only a source of fuel and building blocks, but it is, or should be, one of the great pleasures of life. Nor should meal times be considered just a social exercise. It is well established that eating in a calm and happy environment is conducive to good digestion – and good digestion is the foundation of good health.

IT'S A FAMILY AFFAIR

It is generally acknowledged that there is a trend against meal times as family occasions in the West, and particularly in the UK and USA. Teenagers graze, eat on the run, eat while watching TV, reading or working. These habits start young.

Do we really expect our children to grow up with good table manners and sociable habits if we isolate them and expect them to eat on their own, set the example of eating in front of the TV, or do any of the things that stop eating from being a sociable activity? It is worth making the occasion of eating together a relaxed and enjoyable event. It should be possible to sit down together once a day for a meal – breakfast is usually rushed, but lunch or high tea might be the time to do it. If you cannot organize the whole family, it is at least worth you sitting down while your youngster eats and having a token snack or just a cup of tea with him. At the very least, making a ritual of a family meal once or twice a week or at weekends is a way of keeping the right focus. The idea is to set an example of how it should be – lead from the front. Your child will learn from you about the value of this closeness and will enjoy these times.

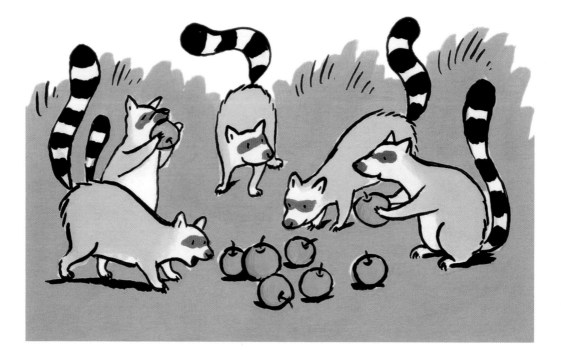

❧ HELP! MY CHILD WON'T EAT ❧

Small children do not have many means of exerting control over their environment. One of the only ways that they can is to accept or refuse food. From a very young age, children become sensitive to their parents' reactions to their behaviour and begin to learn that they can manipulate a situation by their actions.

I have frequently been asked by frustrated parents, who are at their wits' end, what to do about a child who simply refuses to eat, or eats only what is offered as a final bribe – perhaps crisps or biscuits. Here are several steps I suggest undertaking to shift the pattern of behaviour.

1 Stop worrying! Your child will not starve – at some point he will become hungry and eat. This is the hardest thing for most parents, since it is ingrained in most of us to be concerned about children that do not eat – and so many emotions become tied up in this whole issue. If he misses a few meals, he has the physical reserves to compensate for this. Of course, if this goes on for too long and your child is virtually anorexic, you must consult a doctor. However, 99.99% of the time the child begins to eat when the show-down is over.

2 Recognize that children have different appetites, just as adults do. In particular, a lot of children eat more just before a growth spurt, when they fatten up, and are often less hungry when actually going through the growth spurt. Do not let these times become the basis of a bad emotional relationship with food and meal times. Usually, if they do not eat much at one meal, they will compensate at the next one.

3 Do not be tempted to give your child junk food, which he will want to eat, simply in order to get something into him. This lays the ground for all sorts of blackmailing in future, using food as a weapon.

4 If he really does not like a food do not force it on him, but remember that there is a difference between really hating something and simply wanting something else – something which is usually sweeter or saltier.

5 Make sure the food is palatable – you would not want to eat bland mush either. Plan ahead.

6 It is best not to distract your child with a lot of toys and games while eating as poor eaters are often too easily distracted from the main event, which is eating.

7 Whatever you do, do not make a huge fuss if he refuses to eat what you have made as this will almost always spiral into an emotional tug of war. To save your frazzled nerves, having cooked a delicious meal that is now being refused, make sure you have a selection of healthy, quickie options (*see page 104*) that you can offer in preference to unhealthy bribes. If he will not eat the second choice then just leave it – the chances are that he will be hungry at the next snack or meal time.

8 It is quite normal for a child to refuse food when he is unwell. You will notice that the first thing that animals and children do when ill is to stop eating. Adults tend to ignore this natural phenomenon, thinking it necessary to keep your strength up. The complete opposite is true. Digestion is such an energy-charged process that it diverts energy away from the healing process, and the body has more than enough stores for quite a long fast if necessary. So listen to what your child is telling you, if he does not want to eat when sick – do not force him. Keep the liquids up, and when he is hungry he will eat again.

HEALTHY FOOD
A HEALTHY ATTITUDE

Children have likes and dislikes, too. If your child simply does not like a particular food, do not force it on him. You can always try it again later, possibly in a different guise. If you find that your child refuses an entire food group, like meat or green vegetables, do not panic – you can always find another type of food that substitutes for it, or a good way of disguising it (*see page 70 and page 74 for ideas*).

Also, if you start offering a choice of foods, and your youngster refuses what he seems to have wanted only 15 minutes ago, remember that 15 minutes is a long time for a small child. What he wanted then may not be what he wants now. Keep your cool – these things happen and are not necessarily designed to try your patience.

FADS & FUSSPOTS
It is not unusual for a child to go through a phase of eating only a select few foods: baked beans on toast, peanut butter sandwiches or sausages often seem to be favoured. Again, this is not worth worrying about. In the short term it will do no lasting harm and in the long term the chances are fairly good that he will grow out of this phase. If he is not growing out of it, look again at what you are offering him – is it appealing, does it taste good, does it smell good? Look again at the eight steps on page 109. Peer pressure can be very helpful. We know this from a negative point of view – the child who wants sweets because his friend has them – but it can also be used positively. Find a friend or two who eat well and have them for tea a few times to help re-establish better habits with your child.

One mother I know had an interesting experience when her son refused to eat vegetables. Eating with a little friend one day, the friend's (I quote) 'fabulous, friendly, no-nonsense' nanny just knelt down beside him and talked away to him. Every time he opened his mouth to talk she calmly popped in a spoonful of vegetables then, before he had a chance to react, she changed the focus of conversation to something else. I had a very similar situation when my child stopped wanting to swim after a year of enjoying it – a friend broke the negative cycle in a couple of sessions by showing him how much fun it was. An adult other than the parent, whom the child knows and trusts, can often help to reverse less-than-ideal behavioural trends – the parent can be in the room, but preferably out of (blackmailing) vision.

I think there is a vast difference between occasional changes in behaviour and fundamental alterations in patterns of behaviour. The latter are more likely to be an indication that there is some distress. If loss of appetite is a short-term problem and not accompanied by other behavioural changes, I would be fairly relaxed about it – even if it recurs. If, however, it is accompanied by other symptoms, such as sleep disturbance, restlessness, withdrawal, anxiety, irritability, crying more than usual, aches and pains or any other suspicious circumstances or behaviour, then I would be on the alert that a more serious distress or illness is manifesting. For more in-depth information about child behaviour related to food and eating habits see page 185 for some suggested reading.

A REALISTIC APPROACH
We want the best for our children, but life is never ideal. Many things will conspire to ensure that you cannot offer your child the perfect diet all the time. I think that if you can ensure that your child is getting the best food options 70–80% of the time, that is the most that can usually be expected.

The way that I have chosen to handle the subject of eating out with my young son, where the food might not be as healthy as I would like, is to explain that we have a particular way of eating at home and that there is another way of eating elsewhere. He seems to accept this quite happily and enjoys the occasional treat, like a sticky pudding in a restaurant or an ice cream, and then does not pester me for these at home – he associates these with the rituals of a special occasion.

One of the worst things that can happen is to make a great fuss about eating the 'right' foods when not at home – at the expense of making your child self-conscious about food and just desperate to get his hands on the jelly.

There are some easy substitutions that can be made without a young child even noticing, like oatcakes instead of biscuits or curry-flavoured rice crackers instead of crisps, and then there are occasions when you cannot substitute. In this case just go for damage limitation – choose a fruit dessert instead of the triple chocolate fudge whammee.

Children who have a definite allergy and need to avoid a particular food or drink are usually quite sensible if it is explained to them that if they eat that food it will make them unwell. They usually understand this from around the age of two years. Children are frequently better at avoiding the foods in question than the parent is.

EVERYONE HAS AN OPINION

Everyone will have opinions if you ask them. Ask 10 people what you should do about feeding your child; you will get 10 different answers and you will be none the wiser. So the first rule is have the courage of your convictions, and do your own research.

I have been studying the subject for years, and have the benefit of the experience of working with mothers and their children, in addition to my own experience as a mother. Nevertheless, I would urge you to form your own views, based on your own experience, with your own children.

You will also find that everyone you do not ask also has an opinion: your mother and father, parents-in-law, neighbour, health visitor, doctor, absolutely everyone. This is especially the case if, for example, you decide that you do not want your child to have too many sweets, or that your child may have a food allergy, or if you want your child to be a vegetarian or to avoid dairy products as a precautionary measure. 'It didn't hurt me when I was growing up', 'He needs sugar for energy', 'You'll stunt her growth', 'You'll make him an outcast'. These are all unsolicited comments I have heard or been told about.

Of course, it may not hurt to explore the subject – 'granny may well know best'. However, if you have decided on a course of action you feel comfortable with, stick to your guns. He is your child and you will have to deal with the effects of a diet that is not right for him – no one else will. If the disagreement is close to home and you disagree with your partner on the best course of action, sit down together at a quiet moment, get out a big piece of paper and make a list of all the pros and cons of the dietary strategy that is under dispute. The solution will usually work itself out. If it does not, you can agree to adopt one methodology for a given period of time, and then switch course of action for a following period of time. See which suits your child best. Perhaps your child, if he is older, will have some opinions, too. But remember that you are dealing with a child, not an experimental project.

Finally, have alternative strategies if a difficult situation is likely to recur – for instance, the grandparents who always brings sweets and think this is all right because they do not see their grandchild very often. (You, in the meantime, are left with the hyperactive monster to deal with when they go home.) They may need to be persuaded to bring another token of love, such as colouring books that they can actually enjoy with your child. If you think hard enough, you can usually avert most recurring problems. And frankly, the one-off situations that may occur are not too significant in the long run.

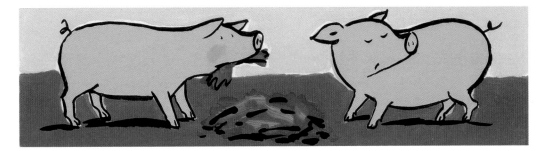

NURSERY
SCHOOL FOOD

I think this deserves a special mention, as the nursery school or at the regular child-minder's is where your child may eat on a regular basis. The first surprise is that a child will quite often behave differently at play-school, eating foods that he normally refuses at home.

Most play-schools are used to dietary problems, in particular allergies and sugar-free diets. First of all, familiarize yourself with a typical week's menu. If it is only a matter of a couple of days a week, it is not worth worrying whether your child is having white rather than wholemeal pasta or white versus brown rice. On the other hand, I normally advise that a particular request be made about avoiding concentrated sources of sugar and any food allergens that you know may cause problems.

Usually most schools can accommodate this and will simply leave out the jelly, fruit yoghurt or cream sauce. They usually provide fruit for desserts and meat and vegetables for main courses. You may want to pack easy snacks like oatcakes, rice crackers, fruit or raisins to fill in the gaps. Again, there is a fine line to be drawn between healthy eating and

making your child feel like an outcast, but up to the age of two or three you can usually get away with it quite easily.

Whatever happens, talk to the teachers or child-minder – they are usually accommodating. If not, shop around and you may find another play-school that is.

BIRTHDAY PARTIES AND OTHER PITFALLS

Unless your child has a wide circle of little friends, these are infrequent occasions. The main problem is sugar. It can cause sleeplessness, hyperactivity and upset tummies – especially if your child is not used to it. My general rule is let them loose on most of the party food; fill them up with what you know they will eat and that which is least damaging – chicken nuggets, little sandwiches, cherry tomatoes, breadsticks, corn chips, raisins, diluted orange juice – by which time they will be too full, or distracted, to really care about the rest. I suggest avoiding the sugary cordials, jelly and brightly coloured chocolate drops or mini-biscuits, but allowing a little

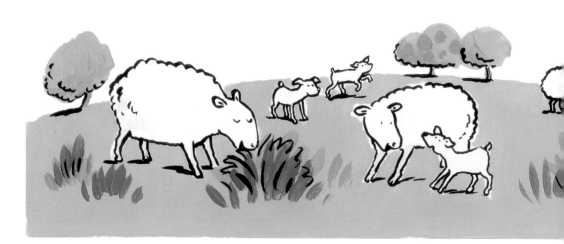

birthday cake (keeping the icing to a minimum). This usually works.

If you are going to a party where you suspect that the food on offer will be way down the health scale, you could always feed your little one before you go to blunt his appetite. I also have to admit that I have been known to cheat and fill up empty crisp packets with sugar-free cornflakes – they sound and crunch the same as the real thing, and none of the children seemed to mind! Of course, if it is you who is throwing the birthday party, you can offer a healthy selection of foods – see page 154.

❧ THE CHOCOLATE QUESTION ❧

Many parents will firmly refuse to let their children have chocolate preferring not to allow a chocoholic to emerge. The addicts among us adults will go to endless lengths to justify our addiction. So what are the pros and cons?

❧ CONS: ❧

Most chocolate for children is sold as milk chocolate and has a very high sugar content. This means that the impact on blood sugar levels is substantial (*see page 62*). This is emphatically not to be recommended for children. Chocolate is also very high in caffeine which is a potent stimulant. The manufacturing process can be questionable, with many additives and colourings.

❧ PROS: ❧

The dark chocolate, preferably with 70% cocoa solids, has very little effect on blood sugar levels, is a source of iron and magnesium and contains significant amounts of phenols (antioxidants), lowering cardiovascular risk. Compared to sweets, chocolate causes less tooth decay. It does, however, have a strong hit of caffeine.

As children do like to be like their peers, I think there is no harm in occasionally grating a little organic 70% cocoa chocolate on top of desserts, or as a topping for a plain wholemeal cake. Fruit cubes dipped in melted chocolate are delicious. I find that a little can go a long way and stops the urgency of wanting something that is forbidden. If you find that your child is sensitive to the caffeine, cut back on this treat.

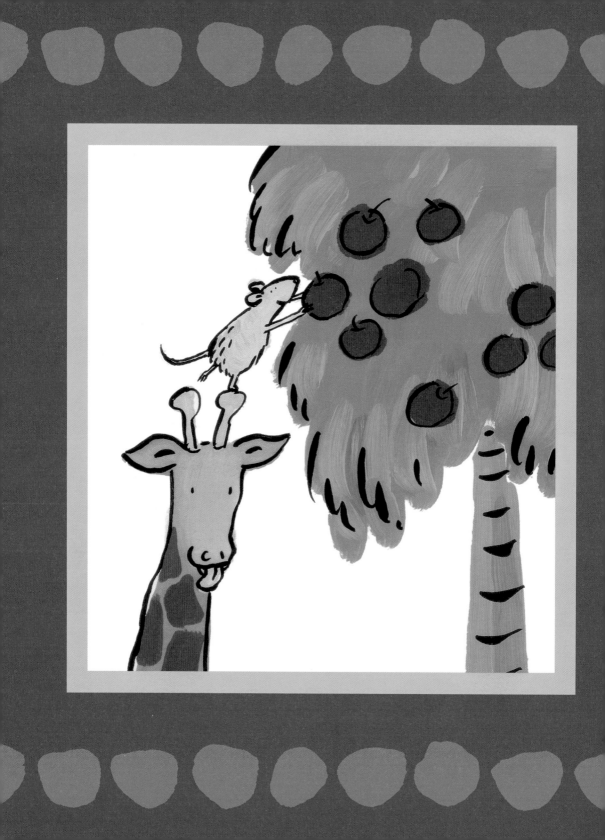

9

SOLUTIONS, NOT PROBLEMS

I f you adopt a positive outlook, it is amazing how you can transform 'problems' into exciting challenges to be overcome. A positive attitude like this is definitely a plus when dealing with children, as the road to healthy adulthood is paved with many 'challenges'. The common problems that are dealt with here can all be viewed as opportunities to increase your understanding – it might not feel like this when you are going through a crisis, but viewing it this way makes the experience more acceptable.

IMMUNITY
FOR LIFE

What can you do to maximize your child's chances in the permanent battle his body is waging against the outside world? The following are some key steps.

Antioxidant status: Make sure your child's antioxidant status is good. Antioxidants are vitamins, minerals and other natural chemicals that fight free radicals (unstable molecules that damage cells). Antioxidants protect because they give up their own molecules to stabilize, or quench, the free radical before it does too much damage. A good supply of antioxidants will do a lot to reduce the harm done by the 10,000 free-radical 'hits' that, it has been estimated, each cell takes every day. Current thinking is that free radicals are at the core of around 80 different diseases, including diabetes, asthma, eye problems and allergies. A diet rich in antioxidants supports immune health.

Antioxidants in the diet come from fresh fruit and vegetables. At least five portions daily are advised – these five portions a day have been shown, in study after study, to be closely linked to reduced risks of cancer and heart disease. Apart from the known antioxidants – vitamins A, C, E and the minerals zinc and selenium – there are other nutrients to think about. The B-vitamins and the minerals chromium and magnesium have an antioxidant effect by balancing energy functioning and so reducing oxidative stress.

There are a whole series of phytonutrients (*see page 72*) and bioflavanoids that have an antioxidant effect. What is interesting about these is that the antioxidants are actually the natural pigments that give fruit and vegetables their colours. So a plateful of colourful food will automatically improve your child's antioxidant status (*see below*).

❧ ANTIOXIDANTS ❧

COLOUR	FOOD EXAMPLES	COMPOUNDS	PROPERTIES
Red	Tomatoes, pink grapefruits watermelons	Lycopene	Antioxidant Anticancer
Orange	Carrots, apricots, papayas, cantaloupes, squashes, mangoes	Beta-carotene and other carotenoids	Anticancer
Yellow	Corn, yellow peppers	Beta-carotene	Anticancer
	Turmeric, cumin Mustard	Curcumin Isothiocyanates	Anticancer Anticancer
Green	Cabbages, Brussels sprouts, kale, broccoli, green beans	Chlorophyll	Magnesium rich, inhibits cancer-causing chemicals
Purple	Blueberries, blackberries red grapes, cherries	Anthocyanidins Proanthocyanidins	Anti-inflammatory Improves collagen formation, good for eyesight and circulation

Optimal bacterial balance: Ensure that the bacterial balance of your child's digestive tract is optimal. Poor bacterial balance is a stress on the immune system as it has to deal with pathogenic bacteria. The most likely sources of poor bowel bacteria balance are bottle-feeding, antibiotics and low fibre in the diet. Symptoms of poor bacterial balance in a child would be excessive wind, regular bouts of diarrhoea or constipation. Additionally, any skin complaint could be an indication, since the skin is an organ of elimination that shows up problems when the bowels are not working as efficiently as they could be. Keep the bacterial balance in good shape by ensuring your child has lots of soluble fibre from fruit, vegetables and grains. If necessary, give your child a specially formulated infant bacterial supplement in powder form in his drink, and certainly do so after using antibiotics (*see page 122*).

Identifying allergies: If you suspect your child suffers from food allergies or intolerances, identify them (*see page 96*) and seek to eliminate them. Any intolerance will tax the immune system, leaving it less free to deal with other immune-related problems.

Plenty of water: Make sure your child drinks enough water. Water helps to keep toxins flushed out, meaning they are not hanging around to add an extra load on the immune system.

Vitamin C: No information about immunity would be complete without a special mention of vitamin C since it is effective on so many levels. Firstly, it is both antiviral and antibacterial. Experiments show that in the laboratory viruses perish in a vitamin C-rich environment. Furthermore, it is essential for building white blood cells, which are the chief soldiers in the immunity army – not enough vitamin C equals not enough white blood cells. If all this were not enough, vitamin C is also imperative for collagen formation. Collagen 'glues' cells together, making them less penetrable to invading organisms and acting as a first line of defence. Finally, vitamin C is not only a powerful antioxidant in its own right but also has the intriguing ability to 'protect' vitamin E (another antioxidant), thereby extending the usage of body stores and reducing dependence on dietary sources. I give my child the extra boost of a good-quality vitamin C powder once or twice a day in his drink.

❧ HEALTHY TEETH ❧

At birth your baby's teeth are fully formed, lying just under the gum surface waiting to come through. So, from a nutritional point of view, the work on the formation of the teeth has already been done before your child was born.

The nutritional needs for healthy teeth are the same as for healthy bones – good amounts of calcium, magnesium, vitamin D, vitamin C, zinc and boron from the diet. (Boron is available from a wide range of vegetables as well as apples, pears, grapes and nuts). The nutritional needs for healthy gums are just as important – vitamin C for connective tissue formation, vitamin A for mucous membrane integrity, zinc, essential fatty acids and a substance we manufacture called coenzyme Q10.

I prefer not to use fluoridated toothpaste as some of it will be swallowed or absorbed across the mucosa of the mouth. The fluoride in sodium fluoride, which is used in most commercial brands of toothpaste, links up very easily with calcium, which is why it is used to strengthen teeth. But in a small child with developing bones, I am uneasy about fluoride that can bind with calcium in bones, effectively 'hardening' them and reducing the turnover of bone tissue, which is vital for proper growth. Getting the balance right with fluoride is very difficult, especially if using fluoridated products in an area where the water is also fluoridated. One part per million is the amount that is recommended to strengthen teeth, while only two parts per million is highly toxic. A sign of excess fluoride is mottling of the teeth – this is irreversible. Fluoride has also been implicated in diseases later in life including osteoporosis, thyroid disease and cancer.

I prefer to use unfluoridated toothpaste or one that uses calcium fluoride – these are available from health food shops. Around the age of two is probably the right time for your child's first dental check-up – be sure to pick a dentist who is child-friendly! Later on, as adult teeth emerge you can ask your dentist to apply a sealant coat to flat tooth surfaces to ensure no cavities develop.

VERY ACTIVE
OR HYPERACTIVE?

In my experience, a well-nourished child on a nutritionally sound diet is a happy and calm child – often boisterous, but not hyperactive. In addition to hyperactivity there is a category called Attention Deficit Disorder (ADD) and the two are often lumped together. ADD will often be treated with a drug called Ritalin, a stimulant which, paradoxically, drugs children into a soporific state.

I believe that nutrition ought to be the first port-of-call for any concerned parent, before resorting to serious drugs to sedate a child. A study published in the *Lancet* concluded that 82% of hyperactive children treated by diet alone improved significantly and one-third of them returned to completely normal behaviour. These results were then confirmed in further studies.

The first questions to ask are: is the child truly hyperactive or just more active than you think is ideal? Does he simply have a shorter-than-usual attention span? Is he looking for attention? Is he bored? He may not be hyperactive at all. A key pointer is to determine whether your child is capable of sitting still for periods of time, possibly playing quietly or concentrating on small, focused tasks. If he does do this on occasions, then he is probably just boisterous the rest of the time. You may find that his energy spurts happen to coincide with times when you are feeling drained of energy making it seem worse than it is. There are many possible contributing factors to hyperactivity, but the following are the main nutritional problems to look out for.

Sugar: Sugar is a likely source of the problem, and frequently this is all that needs to be addressed. It is certainly the one item on which to be non-negotiable if your child is showing signs of hyperactive behaviour. Hyperactivity is often only a reaction to a sudden burst of sugar – watch a tired child go over the top half an hour after a sweet drink and you will see why. Avoid all sources of sugar and refined carbohydrates, and strive to maintain good blood sugar levels (*see page 62*) as much as possible.

Food additives and colourings: These are the next most likely contributory factors. In particular, the yellow colouring, tartrazine, has been implicated in hyperactivity. Avoid all prepackaged foods that may contain such additives.

🖤 SALICYLATES 🖤

Salicylates are naturally occurring chemicals, related to aspirin, which are found in many fruit and some vegetables. They seem to be involved in some children's hyperactivity. The Feingold diet, devised by Dr Ben Feingold, was designed to avoid salicylates and books on the subject are available. If other steps do not work, it is worth investigating this option.

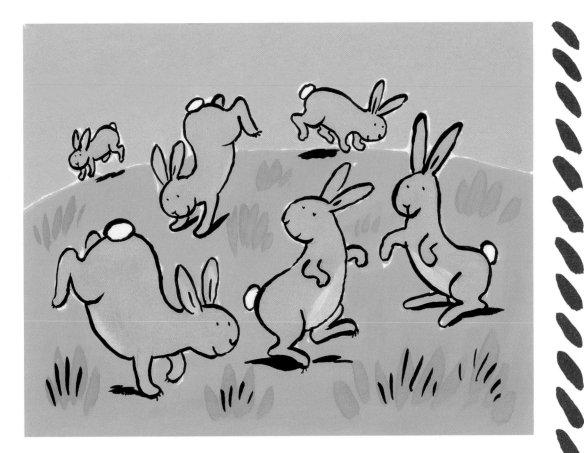

Food sensitivities: Food sensitivities may be involved and wheat, in particular, is often a problem. Other grains should also be suspected. Sometimes other Type I allergies may be involved, for example pollen or animal dander (hair) allergies. A majority of hyperactive children come from families with a history of allergies.

Essential fats: Research shows that the types of fats that have the most pronounced effect on improving hyperactivity are DHA, GLA, EPA and AA – all of which can be found in supplemental form (*see also page 48*). Correcting a child's essential fat status works 60 percent of the time.

Heavy metal toxicity and other problems: Heavy metal toxicity, especially from lead, aluminium or copper, can result in nervous disruption. If you suspect this you should keep pollutants to a minimum (*see page 95*) and possibly consult a nutritional therapist, who can conduct laboratory tests such as a hair mineral analysis to determine if this is the case (*see page 186*). The mineral analysis will also give an indication of other mineral levels that are important for good nerve functioning, including zinc and magnesium levels.

Zinc can also be tested with a sweat test and a red cell magnesium blood test is possible. However, I think that a hair test is less invasive and the latest testing facilities are very accurate. A nutritional therapist can also evaluate, via a specialized urine test, if there are any amino acid imbalances – these play an important role in brain function and can help to rebalance out-of-synch neurotransmitters.

Hyperactive children may need a higher-than-normal protein diet as they metabolize more quickly, but this should be done under supervision in the case of a small child. Thyroid function needs to be considered as the child may have a slightly hyperactive thyroid, and this problem can often be helped by identifying food allergies and cutting out sugar, as mentioned previously.

TOO THIN,
TOO FAT...

Grown-up people come in all shapes and sizes, and so do little people. Wouldn't it be a boring world if we didn't? We know what the average child should be but, remember, your child is not average but unique. His genetics will play a large part in his shape, and he may well take after great-uncle Fred on your mother's side of the family. However, if you are really concerned about your child's weight, below are a few pointers.

TOO THIN

Babies usually lose some of their birth weight in the first two or three weeks of life – a few ounces or so. This is quite normal, but may be a cause for concern to new parents.

Growth usually happens in spurts, and it is normal for toddlers not to put on weight for several weeks before suddenly shooting up. If your child is ill for any length of time, this may also contribute to him being slightly underweight for a while. If it goes on for too long the doctor may diagnose what is known as 'failure to thrive', a term that relates to small children who do not gain height and weight as they should and whose growth is not steady for an extended period of time.

If you are concerned about your child not eating and being underweight, and I must say it is a very rare situation, you may want to consider the following:

❤ Are there any emotional signals being picked up by your child? Loss of appetite can be associated with emotional stress.

❤ Would your child be better off with 'grazing' instead of 'square meals' – or vice versa?

❤ Are you giving too many low-calorie meals? The current low-fat eating trend for adults is not appropriate for children. They need a good amount of calories from fats – not just any fats, but the right sort of fats (*see page 46*).

❤ Is your child being pressurized at meal times? So many negative associations can be built up if the parents are anxious about types of foods, quantities and so on. Do you enjoy meal times, or are they something to be 'got through'? A child takes cues from his parents, positively and negatively.

❤ Is your child being given enough time to eat? It can take up to an hour for a small child to finish a meal.

❤ If the problem is severe and all the medical and psychological advice is not working, it could be worth exploring the nutritional angle more thoroughly. I do not advise attempting to deal with this problem yourself. Consulting a suitably trained nutritionist may help resolve any possible biochemical imbalances that may be involved. For instance, zinc deficiency can be involved in anorexia, as can essential fatty acid deficiency. Another specialized area in the field of nutrition is the use of amino acids in therapy. Some are remarkably effective at restoring neurotransmitter balance in the brain which can, in turn, lead to a resumption of appetite.

TOO FAT

There was a time when the ideal post-war baby was a little round tub with rosy cheeks. We have moved away from this ideal but babies do need to develop fat stores in order to thrive well. It is a question of balance.

Properly nourished children are less likely to get fat as they are nutritionally saturated. You must, of course, look at the genetic aspect as well, although my theory is that we inherit diet as much as genes, predisposing us to the same weight and health problems as our parents. Look at your own diet first. It is really not fair to expect your child to snack on apples and rice cakes, if you are sneaking biscuits and chocolates, is it?

Sometimes the problem starts in babyhood,

especially with bottle-fed babies. This is because of the high levels of saturated fats in cow's milk formulas, and also because some parents are tempted to overfeed their baby with formula milk – almost impossible to do with breast-feeding.

We used to refer to a bit of excess weight in youngsters as 'puppy-fat' and there may be something in that. Children need fat reserves to gear them up for growth spurts, so again it may be wise simply to let them grow out of it.

If you think your child is truly overweight, examine what you are doing and consider the advice in this book. If you are unhappy that your child has an exceptionally sweet tooth and always reaches for the sweets, doughnuts and cakes, I would ask 'Why does he have access to them?' He cannot be going to birthday parties every day! Look at the section 'A Realistic Approach' (*page 110*) and the maxim that 'we eat this way at home and make a few changes when we are out'.

I would balk at putting a small child (or any child or adult for that matter) on a 'diet'. The word diet implies a short-term activity, and usually has negative, calorie-controlled, low-fat connotations. Diets have been shown over and over again not to work – they usually result in the yo-yo syndrome of losing and gaining weight countless times. I would prefer to see long-term changes to eating habits, which encompass the 'right' fats, complex carbohydrates high in pulses, beans, fruit and vegetables. The foods to keep to a minimum are sugars, refined carbohydrates, red meat, saturated or hydrogenated fats, fried foods, packaged or processed foods and excess fruit juices.

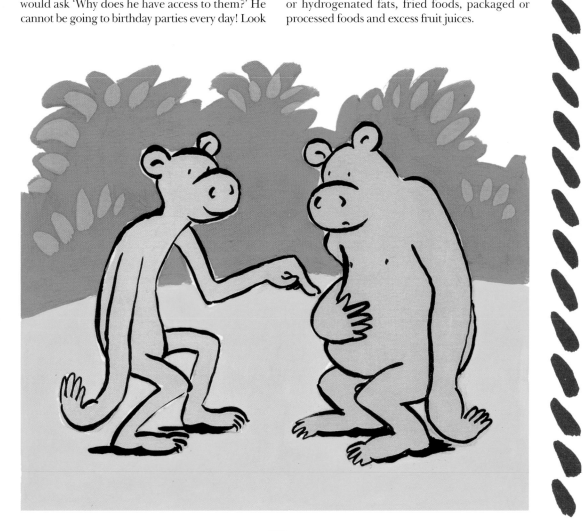

REMEDIES
FOR COMMON
AILMENTS

Comparing notes at play-groups, it immediately becomes apparent that many children suffer from the same illnesses over and over again. Some are minor, some are quite nasty. Either way it is always distressing for the child, and equally so for the parent to stand by and see their child in discomfort.

There are many things we can do both to alleviate the immediate distress, and also to avoid recurrence – or even to avoid the problem in the first place.

The information here is designed to be used with discretion. A parent needs always be vigilant in case the problem is getting out of control and, if concerned, always call in a doctor – it is not worth taking a risk.

ANTIBIOTICS

Antibiotics are, of course, not an ailment. I have simply included them on this list because so many children are given courses of antibiotics early in life – sometimes justifiably, and sometimes not. Antibiotics can be useful, even life-saving, if used selectively. Like many parents I am very fussy about subjecting my child to these drugs. Overuse can lead to resistance later in life, a suppressed immune system and, more immediately, an imbalance in the bowel bacteria that are so important to overall health (*see page 18*). Alarming statistics have also emerged showing that 'clusters' of meningitis are occurring in areas where there is overuse of antibiotics in the community.

If you do have to give your child antibiotics, I strongly suggest that you replace the 'good' bacteria that would have been swept out with the pathogenic bacteria. A good infant formulation, Bifido Infantis, is supplied by Biocare (*see page 186*). It can be dissolved in a little water and fed to small babies in bottles, on a teaspoon or through a dropper, when the course of antibiotics has been completed.

If you and your doctor decide that the illness is not serious enough to warrant antibiotics there are alternative, natural antibacterials: garlic, propolis, manuka honey, aloe vera juice, tea tree oil and grapefruit seed extract (applied diluted, topically only for children – and not near the eyes). See page 186 for suppliers of these products and follow the manufacturers' instructions.

ASTHMA

This can be a serious condition and must be addressed. The current medical practice is to treat it quite heavy-handedly with steroids, which does seem to have a better prognosis – although I would be concerned about the long-term impact on the immune system in adulthood. Asthma tends to run in families that are called 'atopic' – in other words they are genetically susceptible to allergic reactions such as asthma, eczema and migraines. Quite often we are told that children 'will grow out of it' and indeed, superficially this does seem to happen. There is a growing incidence of asthma – one in ten children are affected – and it is presumed that this is due to increased pollution levels. The main triggers, as opposed to the underlying factors, are usually house dust mite droppings, animal hair, changes in air temperature, allergies, pollution, infections, stress and medicines. It seems obvious that the situation would be worse in big cities, but some rural areas have a much higher count, probably because there is so much agricultural crop spray in the air.

There are a couple of important aspects to look out for. Firstly, there is quite frequently misdiagnosis of this condition in small children – maybe because some doctors do not have enough time to consider all the factors. I have known several children to be treated for asthma with steroids, when all they had was an upper-respiratory tract infection. If you are concerned, it is worth getting a second opinion. Secondly, the 'triggers' are often just that – the straw that breaks the camel's back. It is important to look for underlying factors, such as pollution, diet and nutrient levels. As to a child 'growing out of the condition', I believe that, in an attempt to maintain equilibrium the body adapts and the symptoms are alleviated – only to appear years later in a different form: migraines, irritable bowel syndrome, chronic fatigue, for example.

You will find that I constantly refer to wheat and dairy allergies and essential fatty acid deficiencies. This is because they are so widespread and may lead to different health problems from child to child – if they are implicated. In relation to asthma, dairy products – especially the full fat type – are known to be pro-inflammatory. Wheat can have the effect of triggering histamine. If you are still breast-feeding, remember that wheat or dairy products in the mother's diet can have just as much of an effect as introducing these foods directly into a child's diet. Essential fats, especially the omega-3 fish oils, have a beneficial bronchio-dilatory effect. However it is necessary to take care with the omega-6 fats such as evening primrose oil, as in excess they can encourage inflammation. It is important to get a good balance between the two types of fats. (It is for the same physiological reason that asthmatics are unable to tolerate aspirin). GLA and EPA fats (*see page 48*) for asthmatics may be particularly important as those with an atopic (genetic) tendency often do not convert the essential fats in their bodies into the anti-inflammatory substances, called prostaglandins, as efficiently as other people.

Other considerations for asthmatics are good fluid levels and making sure they have enough zinc (found in ground seeds) and beta-carotene (found in carrot juice).

To keep house dust mites to a minimum make sure that bedding is kept scrupulously clean and, preferably, remove carpets in favour of wood, linoleum or tiled flooring. For more information on specialist equipment for reducing the allergy potential of your home see the addresses on page 184.

COLIC

The worst time for colic is between the ages of two and five months. There are several very useful steps to take to minimize colic. The first thing to do is to exclude wheat and dairy if they are being fed to a child, or to exclude them from the mother's diet if breast-feeding. Onions and garlic can also have an effect. One study showed that 70% of bottle-fed infants with colic improved when they were moved on to formula feeds that did not contain cow's milk protein.

It is important to feed from one breast at each feed from beginning to end. Breast milk is delivered as first and main courses. The initial flow is quite thin and has a high protein and milk sugar content – possibly to alleviate immediate hunger – and the next stage is quite thick and fatty to sustain for a bit longer. If the baby is switched between breasts all they get is the thin sugary milk which makes colic worse, since more lactose (milk sugar) reaches the bowel where it then ferments.

Colic may be an indication of lactose intolerance if the child is being bottle-fed. Adding lactose enzymes to bottle milk can resolve this. Corn syrup in formulas can also cause a problem. One cow's milk Omnescomfort is lactose reduced and includes 'Pre-biotics' and reduces discomfort very well.

After feeding, burp your baby and then lay him on his right side so that trapped wind will not be forced into his intestines. Baby massage can also help. It may also help if you do not feed more frequently than every two hours and give unsweetened, cooled camomile tea half an hour before a milk feed. Other teas to try, one at a time, are fennel seed, dill seed or mint – add half a teaspoon of whichever herb you are trying to a cup of boiling water, then cool it to room temperature; strain it and give one to three teaspoons by dropper or on a spoon. Adding infant bacteria (*see suppliers, page 186*) to your baby's feed or water may also help with colic.

CONSTIPATION

It is agonizing to see a little baby or toddler straining to do a poo and being really uncomfortable. Also, if this discomfort goes on for too long, the child can begin to associate pain with going to the toilet, and can deliberately try not to go – making the vicious cycle worse. Ideally, small children, who have very short digestive tracts compared to adults, should go about twice a day. If your child is constipated, consider the following. Is he getting enough liquids to keep the stools soft? Is there enough fibre in his diet, especially the fibre found in fruit, vegetables, rice and oats? (You should never give a small child wheat bran as a fibre source since it relieves constipation only by irritating the gut wall, which is undesirable.) Is he intolerant to any food, especially milk/dairy (very common) or wheat, or the other grains? Is he emotionally distressed? If your child is constipated, a useful measure to try is to mix a couple of teaspoons of olive oil in with his food – olive oil increases peristalsis (movement) of the digestive tract quite remarkably.

DIARRHOEA

This can be quite dangerous in a small child if it goes on for too long, as children can become seriously dehydrated. If you think this may be happening, consult your doctor, who will probably suggest an electrolyte solution. Most of the time diarrhoea is a sign that the body needs to evacuate something which is causing an irritation. The most obvious possibility to consider is some kind of food poisoning – this may be accompanied by vomiting. It is often the case that a food sensitivity is to blame, and it is frequently the foods that are eaten most regularly which cause the trouble. Culprits can include wheat and dairy products (yes again!), other grains such as rye or oats, soya milk, citrus fruit, especially oranges, and any other food that is eaten too frequently. Foods that can help get rid of diarrhoea are brown rice and live yoghurt.

ECZEMA

The advice here is similar to that for asthma, since they share many of the same dietary risk factors. Some babies are covered from head to foot in eczema, which is sad because much can be done to prevent it.

Once again consider allergies: wheat and other grains such as oats, rye, corn and barley, all dairy products, soya products and citrus fruit are top of the list. It is important to keep saturated fats from meat and dairy to a bare minimum since they can cause inflammatory flare-ups. The GLA and EPA derivatives of essential fats (see page 48) could be very important. Some eczema sufferers seem not to be able to make the conversion of essential fats into the compounds the body uses to bring down inflammation. By using GLA (found in evening primrose oil) and EPA (found in oily fish) you skip this conversion step. Zinc (found in ground seeds) and vitamin A (found in carrot juice) are helpful, as is making sure water intake is kept up.

You can also try piercing evening primrose oil and vitamin E gelatine capsules and gently rubbing them directly on to the affected areas – they are absorbed quite well through the skin. One or two capsules a day should be enough.

GLUE EAR

This is a build-up of sticky fluid in the middle ear, usually as a result of repeated infections or allergy, and its correct term is otitis media. The biggest culprits here are dairy produce and too much sugar. I would immediately suggest that any child with glue ear avoids milk and cheese totally. Glue ear is on the increase: 17 out of 20 children under the age of 6 have experienced this problem, and the usual course of treatment is antibiotics. If it gets bad enough, the next stage is grommets in the ear canal. Yet glue ear can be mostly avoided by cutting out dairy products and sugar; if this does not produce results, suspect other allergens. Your child's hearing should always be checked a few weeks after an ear infection.

HAY FEVER

Hay fever does not usually develop in very small children, but you may notice a seasonal tendency to sneezing and watery, itchy eyes. I would consider wheat as a likely culprit, since wheat is a member of the grass family, and can increase the 'load', leading to hay fever symptoms. It is a good idea to avoid wheat for six weeks or so to see if it helps. You may also suspect oats and rye if avoiding wheat does not do the trick.

Histamine is the body chemical that triggers hay fever symptoms and two nutrients work together to help get rid of histamine: calcium helps to release the histamine from the mast cells and vitamin C detoxifies the histamine and carries it out of the body.

MUCUS

Many small children, especially if they go to play-group, have a permanently runny nose. Clear mucus is normal, as they are building up their immunity to a vast number of viruses, and the problem usually decreases with age. The naturopathic attitude to mucus is that it is a natural cleansing mechanism. However, if it seems that the mucus is too thick or is going on for too long, or that there is excessive mucus in the nasal passages, without a cold or infection, you can suspect an allergy. The potential culprit list includes all dairy products, wheat and other grains and soya products. Ensuring good levels of water intake helps to keep your baby's system clear of toxic build-up and reduces the need to excrete toxins via mucus. The enzyme found in pineapples, called bromelin, has been shown to help reduce mucus as a result of allergic responses.

NAPPY RASH

Some people seem to think that nappy rash is normal and I have seen children with almost permanently sore bottoms. It is not normal and can be avoided. Cleanliness is important – make sure that nappies are changed regularly and that your baby is not allergic to the wipes or creams by using cotton balls and water for a period of time. Give your baby's bottom an airing from time to time – leave off the nappy for a while if you can. You may notice that nappy rash seems to occur when stool consistency is not normal, indicating that there may be a component of the diet that is not helping. Ensuring that all the skin nutrients are in the baby's diet in good amounts is important, for example zinc, vitamin A, vitamin C and the essential fats. A good soothing alternative to talcum powder is green clay which has anti-inflammatory properties (*see page 186 for supplier*).

VOMITING

Some babies are 'sicky' babies and their parents seem constantly to have wet patches on their shoulders. This seems to me to occur more frequently with bottle-fed babies – formula milk is not as digestible as mother's milk for young babies. I would switch to other formulas or try to reinstate breast-feeding. Projectile vomiting is another matter and could indicate something more serious. If this happens once or twice, it probably indicates an infection or allergy. If it goes on it may be more serious. In either case contact your doctor as dehydration could swiftly follow.

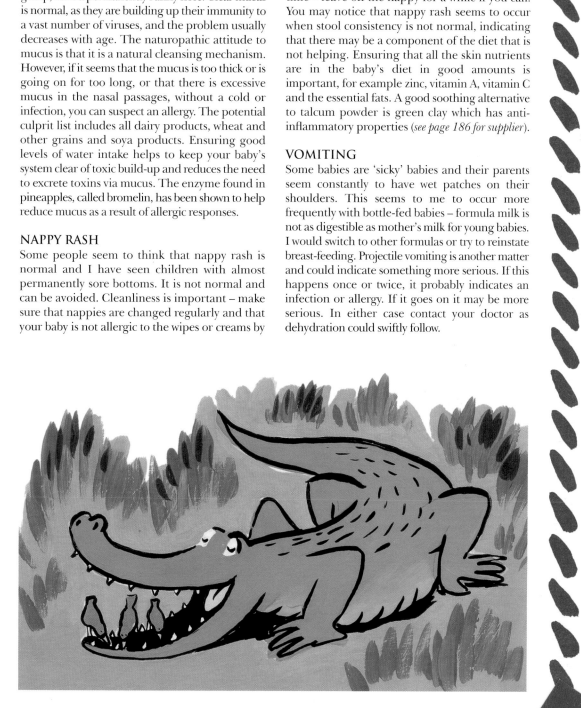

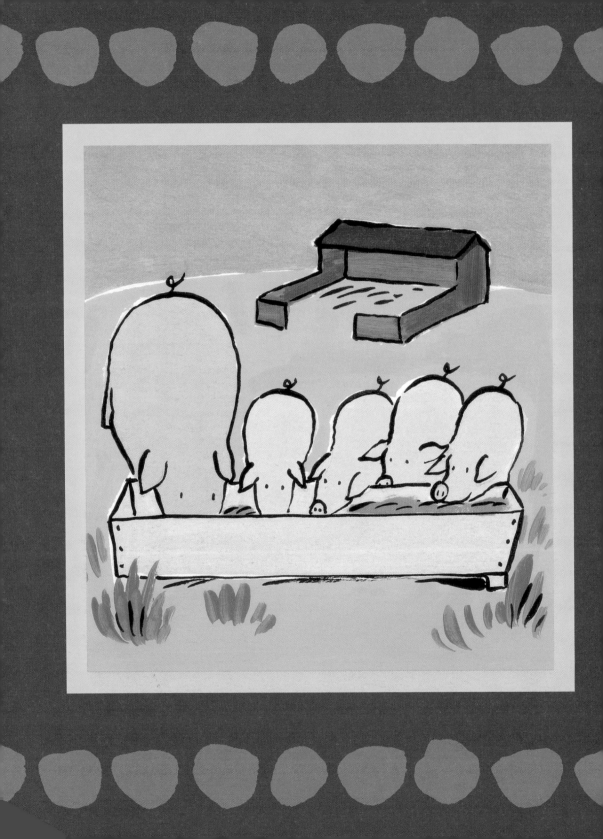

10

MEAL PLANNERS & RECIPES

~~~~~~~~~~~~~~~~

I prefer to spend as little time as possible in the kitchen, and as much time as possible pursuing other interests, not least being with my family. With this in mind, Susan Herrmann Loomis has designed the recipes to be simple to follow with as little preparation time as possible, while still producing varied and delicious results. Recipes have also been planned as meals to be eaten by the whole family, or to be suitable for freezing in child-size portions.

HOW TO USE
THIS SECTION

The recipes have been designed to fit in with the meal planners and have generally kept the exposure to dairy produce and gluten grains to a minimum, while still offering recipes that are delicious and straightforward.

We have delberately not included a lot of esoteric health-food ingredients that may be difficult to find in the shops. Healthy eating is a state of mind, not a difficult shopping trip. But if you cannot find the ingredient in your supermarket, investigate your local health food shop or ethnic food shops, or contact one of the suppliers listed at the back of this book.

The meal planners have been organized by age to help you introduce foods in a manner that is least likely to provoke allergies, food intolerances or sensitivities as discussed in previous sections of this book. They have also been designed to show you how simple it is feed your child a wide variety of foods, and in so doing, provide a wide range of nutrients. Meal Planner entries marked with an asterisk indicate that the recipe is given in this chapter, see the Recipe Index for page numbers.

If you are accustomed to relying on such staples as pasta or bread, you may feel that the programme is restrictive, but I urge you to look at the situation with different eyes. Take it slowly, making a few changes at a time and it will soon become second nature. It is worth a bit of extra effort in the beginning, for the sake of your child's health.

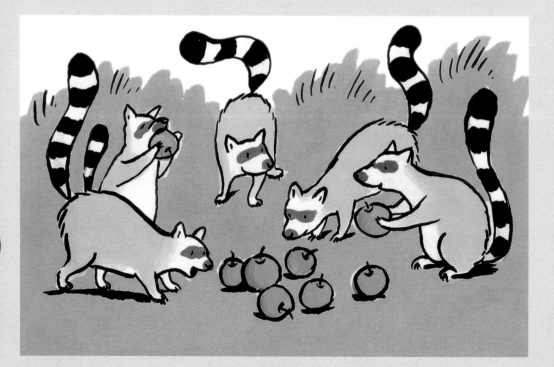

4 - 6 MONTHS

The texture of the food should be a semi-liquid purée with no lumps or strings and salt should not be added. You can also offer water or cooled camomile tea in between feeds. Feed on demand if you prefer, but you may want to begin establishing a routine at around this age. If you are unsure how to start, prepare each of the purées on pages 130-33 and freeze in ice-cube portions. They must be reheated thoroughly. Follow the planners, and feed in single ice cube portions, increasing quantities gradually and adding more foods as listed below.

FOODS TO INTRODUCE:
Introduce foods one by one, being alert to any reactions.

Vegetables: Cook all vegetables until tender prior to liquidizing. The exception is ripe avocado, which can be served raw after your child has been on solids for about 4 weeks. Use any of the following either singly or in combination: Sweet potato, butternut squash, parsnip, carrot, swede, yam, pumpkin, courgette*, cauliflower, broccoli*, green beans*, mangetouts, onion*, artichoke hearts, mushrooms, beetroot*, turnip*, breadfruit, plantain (*may taste better in combination with other vegetables).

Fruits: All skins should be removed. Use any of the following, either singly or in combination: Banana, apples (cooked, or raw and blended), apricot, peach, nectarines, plums, pear, papaya, mango, melon, dried apricots, prunes.

Grains: Brown rice, millet, quinoa.

Pulses: Red Lentils, peas, flageolets.

Fats: One teaspoon a day of cold-pressed flax, sunflower or safflower oil mixed with solids.

Weeks 1 & 2

BREAKFAST
Breast or bottle

MID MORNING
Breast or bottle

LUNCH
Breast or bottle
Single vegetable
(Add baby rice from Week 2)

MID AFTERNOON
Breast or bottle

TEA TIME
Breast or bottle
(Single fruit from Week 2)

BED TIME
Breast or bottle

Weeks 3 & 4

BREAKFAST
Breast or bottle
Single Fruit & Brown Rice Purée*
or Quinoa-Millet Porridge*

MID MORNING
Breast or bottle

LUNCH
Breast or bottle
Single Vegetable with
Lentil* or Flageolet* Purée

MID AFTERNOON
Breast or bottle

TEA TIME
Breast or bottle
Mixed Vegetable & Single Fruit

BED TIME
Breast or bottle

APPLE PURÉE

The cooking time of the apples will vary depending on their variety and freshness.

MAKES ABOUT 600ML/1 PINT
OR 40 CUBES

1kg/2lb apples, cored, peeled and cut into small chunks
125ml/4fl oz filtered water

Place the apples and water in a medium, heavy-bottomed saucepan. Cover and cook over medium heat until the apples are tender and can be easily broken apart with a wooden spoon, about 35 minutes. Remove from the heat and let cool. Purée in a food processor or food mill.

Freeze the purée in ice-cube trays. When the cubes have frozen, store in air-tight freezer safe containers. The cubes will keep for about 2 months.

FRESH APRICOT PURÉE

The same method can be used for nectarines and peaches, but peaches should be peeled.

MAKES ABOUT 125ML/4FL OZ
OR 8 CUBES

500g/1lb whole fresh, ripe apricots

Place the apricots in a steamer set over boiling water, cover and steam until they are tender through, 7–9 minutes. Remove the steamer from the pan and let the apricots stand until they are cool enough to handle.

Remove the stones from the apricots, then purée the fruit in a food processor or food mill.

Freeze the purée in ice-cube trays. When the cubes have frozen, store in air-tight freezer safe containers. The cubes will keep for about 2 months.

CARROT PURÉE

MAKES ABOUT 250ML/8FL OZ
OR 16 CUBES

*500g/1lb carrots, trimmed, peeled
and coarsely chopped*

*To make a richer treat stir in some live yoghurt and ground fresh
nuts for older children.*

Place the carrots in a steamer basket set over boiling water, cover
and steam until they are tender through, 30–35 minutes.
Transfer the carrots to a food processor or food mill and purée.
Cool the purée to room temperature.
Freeze the purée in ice-cube trays. When the cubes have frozen,
store in air-tight freezer safe containers. The cubes will keep for
about 2 months.

PARSNIP PURÉE
Use the same quantity of peeled and sliced parsnips and steam, as
above, for 30–35 minutes. Purée and freeze as above.

DRIED APRICOT PURÉE

MAKES ABOUT 185ML/6FL OZ
OR 12 CUBES

*250g/8oz dried apricots
125ml/4fl oz water*

*Dried apricots deliver a good measure of iron and carotenoids.
Unsulphured apricots are best.*

Place the apricots and water in a small, heavy-bottomed saucepan
over medium heat. Cover and bring the liquid to a boil. Reduce the
heat so the water is simmering and cook until the apricots have
absorbed all the water and softened substantially, 15–20 minutes.
Check the apricots occasionally to be sure they're not sticking to the
bottom of the pan.
Remove the pan from the heat, transfer the apricots to a food
processor or food mill and purée. Let cool, then freeze in ice-cube
trays. When the cubes have frozen, store in air-tight freezer safe
containers. The cubes will keep for about 2 months.

LENTIL PURÉE

MAKES ABOUT 500ML/16FL OZ
OR 32 CUBES

200g/7oz tiny red lentils
400ml/14fl oz filtered water

This is a delicious, versatile and nutritious staple – no household with babies should be without a few cubes in the freezer at all times.

Place the lentils and water in a medium, heavy-bottomed saucepan and bring to a boil over medium-high heat. Cover, reduce the heat so the liquid is boiling gently and cook until the lentils are tender and form a purée when stirred with a wooden spoon. Check the lentils occasionally to be sure there is enough water and that they're not sticking to the bottom of the pan. The lentils will take about 14 minutes to cook through.

Remove the lentils from the heat and stir vigorously with a wooden spoon to make a purée. It will not be perfectly smooth, but will be a very appealing, homogenous texture. Let cool. When the purée has cooled, freeze it in ice-cube trays. When the cubes have frozen, store in air-tight freezer safe containers. The cubes will keep for about 2 months.

PURÉED FLAGEOLETS

MAKES ABOUT 500ML/16FL OZ
OR 32 CUBES

1 large can (800g/26oz) cooked
flageolets without salt,
drained and well rinsed

Red kidney beans, white beans or black-eyed beans can be prepared in the same way for babies who have been on solids for four weeks.

Place the flageolets in a food processor or food mill and purée until they are completely smooth.

Freeze the purée in ice-cube trays. When the cubes have frozen, store in air-tight freezer safe containers. The cubes will keep for about 2 months.

PUMPKIN PURÉE

MAKES ABOUT 500ML/16FL OZ
OR 32 CUBES

1 large chunk of pumpkin
(1–1.5kg/2–3 lb), or the
equivalent of butternut or other
squash, seeded, peeled and cut
into 5cm/2in squares

Naturally sweet, babies take to pumpkin and all other squash readily, and they also deliver a range of anti-oxidants and minerals.

Place the squash in a steamer basket set over boiling water, cover and steam until it is tender through, 15–30 minutes depending on the variety of squash. Remove from the steamer and let cool slightly, then purée in a food processor or food mill.

When the purée is cool, freeze it in ice-cube trays. When they are frozen, store in air-tight freezer safe containers. The cubes will keep for about 2 months.

PEA PURÉE
• • • • • • • • • • • • • •

MAKES ABOUT 250ML/8FL OZ
OR 16 CUBES

250g/8oz fresh or frozen peas
125ml/4fl oz filtered water

Peas give a whopping 9 grams of fibre per cupful and are a rich source of iron. A sprig of mint adds to the flavour.

Place the peas and water in a small saucepan, cover and bring to a boil over medium heat. Cook until the peas are tender, about 7 minutes. Remove from the heat and drain the peas, saving any residual cooking liquid.
Purée the peas in a food processor or food mill, adding the cooking liquid and additional water if necessary to make a smooth purée. Let cool.
When the purée is cool, freeze in ice-cube trays. When the cubes have frozen, store in air-tight freezer safe containers. The cubes will keep for about 2 months.

BROWN RICE PURÉE
• •

MAKES ABOUT 500ML/16FL OZ
OR 32 CUBES

180g/6oz brown rice
750ml/1¼ pints filtered water

This is a healthier alternative to shop-bought baby rice, and it can be used for both sweet and savoury dishes.

Place the rice and water in a medium saucepan, cover and bring to a boil over medium-high heat. Reduce the heat so the liquid is simmering nicely and cook until the rice is tender through, checking once or twice to be sure it isn't sticking.
Remove the rice from the heat and let it cool slightly. Transfer to a food processor or food mill and purée, adding 1–2 tbsp filtered water if necessary to obtain a purée that isn't too thick.
When the rice purée has cooled, freeze it in ice-cube trays. When the cubes have frozen, store in air-tight freezer safe containers. The cubes will keep for about 2 months.

SWEET POTATO PURÉE
• •

MAKES ABOUT 250ML/8FL OZ
OR 16 CUBES

500g/1lb sweet potato,
*   cut into 5cm/2in cubes*

Sweet potatoes are particularly fibre rich and help to stabilize blood sugar.

Place the sweet potato in a steamer basket set over boiling water, cover, and steam until it is tender through, about 15 minutes. Remove the steamer from the pan, transfer the sweet potato to a food processor or food mill and purée. Cool to room temperature. When the purée has cooled, freeze it in ice-cube trays. When the cubes have frozen, store in air-tight freezer safe containers. The cubes will keep for about 2 months.

6 - 9 MONTHS

CONTINUE WITH BREAST OR FORMULA MILK. Breast-fed babies may need a top up of iron in their diet, see page 56 for dietary sources. Gradually increase to three meals a day; serving size will depend on your child's appetite. Salt should still not be added and sweetness can be derived from fruits, fresh fruit juices or blackstrap molasses. The texture of the food should be mashed, puréed or very finely minced. Teeth may start to appear so your baby may enjoy carrot sticks or apple slices to gnaw at (do not leave unattended in case of choking). If the meal planner suggestions do not satisfy your baby, you could also offer some mashed or puréed fresh fruit for dessert.

FOODS TO INTRODUCE:

Introduce foods one by one, being alert to any reactions.

Meat: Oily fish (salmon, tuna, mackerel, sardines), poultry, game and other red meats can be added in in small quantities.

Pulses: Black-eye beans, kidney beans (canned or very well cooked), brown lentils, haricot beans, cannellini beans, mung beans, sprouted pulses and bean sprouts (not sprouted seeds), broad or fava beans (without skins), pinto beans.

Juices: Freshly made juices can be offered with meals (on their own they can promote tooth decay). Exclude citrus juices, but experiment with apple, carrot, pear, melon and others. Make sure there are no seeds, pips or skin, and dilute 50/50 with water.

Fats: Egg yolks. Increase to two teaspoons a day of cold-pressed oils such as flax, walnut, sunflower or safflower and continue this for life.

Seeds: Coconut

Grains: Buckwheat

Menu 1

BREAKFAST
Breakfast Rice*
Breast or bottle

MID MORNING
Breast or bottle

LUNCH
Mashed Avocado or Vegetable Purée
Water

MID AFTERNOON
Breast or bottle

TEA TIME
Lentil Purée*
Fresh Fruit Purée
Water

BED TIME
Breast or bottle

Menu 4

BREAKFAST
Quinoa-Millet Porridge*
Breast or bottle

MID MORNING
Breast or bottle

LUNCH
Pea* & Cabbage Purée with mashed cooked egg yolk
Water

MID AFTERNOON
Breast or bottle

TEA TIME
Sweet Potato*, Leek & Parsnip* Purée
Water

BED TIME
Breast or bottle

Menu 2
• • • • • • • • •

BREAKFAST
Baby Rice & Fruit Purée
Breast or bottle

MID MORNING
Breast or bottle

LUNCH
Flageolet* & Carrot* Purées
Water

MID AFTERNOON
Breast or bottle

TEA TIME
Quinoa* & Mashed Banana
Water

BED TIME
Breast or bottle

Menu 3
• • • • • • • • •

BREAKFAST
Red Lentil Purée* with
Apple Purée*
Breast or bottle

MID MORNING
Breast or bottle

LUNCH
Salmon with Lentil* &
Carrot* Purée
Water

MID AFTERNOON
Breast or bottle

TEA TIME
Vegetable & Brown Rice Purée*
Water

BED TIME
Breast or bottle

Menu 5
• • • • • • • • •

BREAKFAST
Brown Rice* & Mushroom Purée
Breast or bottle

MID MORNING
Breast or bottle

LUNCH
Baked Mackerel with Apple &
Sweet Potato* Purée
Water

MID AFTERNOON
Breast or bottle

TEA TIME
Vegetable & Butter Bean Purée
Water

BED TIME
Breast or bottle

Menu 6
• • • • • • • • •

BREAKFAST
Millet Porridge* & Dried
Apricot* Purée
Breast or bottle

MID MORNING
Breast or bottle

LUNCH
Mashed Avocado
or Banana
Water

MID AFTERNOON
Breast or bottle

TEA TIME
Cannellini Bean Purée* with
Golden Cauliflower Sauce*
Water

BED TIME
Breast or bottle

Breakfast Ideas

THERE ARE MANY ALTERNATIVES TO shop-bought baby rice when you begin to wean your child. Having said this, you may find it handy to have a selection of baby rice and other commercially prepared cereals and jars to hand – see page 36 and 102 for guidelines on acceptable options.

4-6 MONTHS
Because of its smooth consistency, start with baby rice. Once your child is accustomed to solids, move on to brown rice, millet and quinoa. Use the brown rice purée cubes you have in the freezer (*see page 133*) as your basic breakfast staple. Simply defrost, dilute with breast or formula milk and mix with a fruit purée: apple, papaya, mashed banana or any of the fruits listed on page 134. Quinoa and millet flakes are also good (see recipe opposite). They are slightly bitter but this is easily remedied by mixing with mashed ripe banana or fruit purée. Cooked puréed porridges can be frozen in ice-cube trays; additional liquid may be needed to defrost.

6-9 MONTHS
The same still applies but, depending on your child, you may want to offer a coarser texture. You can also begin adding unsweetened flaked coconut, or use unsweetened coconut milk, mixed 50/50 with breast or formula milk. You could also begin offering savoury breakfast options. Try brown rice purée mixed with cooked egg yolk and mushrooms that have been sautéed and puréed. As a bread alternative, try blinis made with buckwheat flour. These can be made in batches, frozen and popped in the toaster to defrost.

9-12 MONTHS
Continue as before, but move on to coarser textures as appropriate for your child. You can now begin adding some plain 'live' yoghurt and cottage cheese in addition to the milk. Grains can be expanded to include oats, rye and barley, and fruits can include berries. It's a good idea to introduce 100% rye bread and crackers now as toddlers do not take to unfamiliar strong tastes as readily as babies. Savoury mixtures can still be made with a rice base, perhaps with the addition of some mashed, cooked organic liver or some finely chopped smoked salmon trimmings.

12-15 MONTHS
By now, breakfast can be almost the same as for adults – it all depends on the chewing ability of your child. Vegetarian sausages (occasionally) and tomatoes can be introduced at this age, so the best standby a tired parent can ask for – baked beans – can become part of the morning ritual. Well-cooked omelettes with any number of fillings are great and little hands can feed themselves if you offer bite-size pieces.

15-24 MONTHS
If you have not yet introduced finely ground seeds and nuts to your child's diet, now is the time, and these can be sprinkled – 1–2 teaspoons or so – over cereal is ideal.

Cheese can now be used but I recommend goat's and sheep's milk cheeses over cow's milk. Finally, wholewheat toast can be introduced, with nut butters and 100% fruit spreads. Try to vary the grains in the breads you offer.

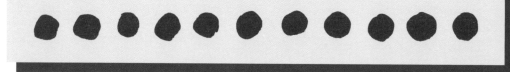

QUINOA-MILLET PORRIDGE

2-3 SERVINGS

30g/1oz quinoa flakes
125ml/4fl oz milk or milk substitute
2 tsp millet flakes
Unsweetened apple juice (optional)
2 cubes dried apricot purée (see
    page 131) or ½ ripe banana,
    mashed

Leftovers can be frozen in airtight containers; you may need to dilute with additional milk, apple juice or boiled filtered water when defrosting. This recipe is suitable from 4-6 months. As your child gets older, ingredients such as oats, ground almonds or sunflower seeds, and coconut can be added (see page 96).

Combine the quinoa flakes and milk in a small saucepan and bring to a boil over low heat. Add more milk if necessary and stir in the millet flakes. Remove from the heat and transfer to a food processor. Process until smooth, adding more milk or apple juice as necessary to thin. Transfer about one-third to a serving bowl, stir in the apricot purée or banana. Test the temperature before serving.

RICE & BARLEY MUESLI

2-3 SERVINGS

30g/1oz barley flakes
30g/1oz rice flakes
125ml/4fl oz milk or milk
    substitute
2 tbsp raisins, diced
2–3 dried apricots, diced
2 tbsp unsweetened flaked
    coconut (optional)

Barley and rice flakes have a tough consistency so this will need to be puréed even for older children. This recipe is suitable from nine months.

Combine the barley and rice flakes and milk in a small saucepan and bring to a boil over low heat. Add more milk if the mixture is too thick. Stir in the raisins, apricots and coconut if using and cook, stirring, for 1 minute. Remove from the heat and transfer to a food processor. Process until smooth, adding more milk as necessary to thin. Test the temperature before serving.

BREAKFAST RICE

1 SERVING

2–4 tbsp Brown Rice Purée (see
    page 133)
½ banana, mashed
4 tbsp apple purée or ¼ peeled,
    grated fresh apple
1 date, stoned and diced
    (optional)
Pinch of ground cinnamon
    (optional)
Warm milk or milk substitute, to
    serve

Keep cubes of brown rice purée in the freezer and this will be a cinch to prepare. For older children, replace the purée with cooked brown rice and serve with coconut milk (from 6 months).

Combine all the ingredients except the milk in a serving bowl and mix. Stir in the milk gradually until the cereal is the desired consistency for your child. Sprinkle with cinnamon if using and serve.

9 - 12 MONTHS

ONTINUE WITH BREAST OR FORMULA MILK. This will still make up a significant part of your child's nutritional requirements and he needs about one pint a day. Solid foods will begin to be the focus of meals and if your child does not seem to have an appetite, you may need to make sure that he is not getting more than a pint of milk a day as this may blunt his appetite. Some grated or coarse lumps can be introduced from around 9 months, taking care to avoid foods that pose an increased risk of choking, such as whole nuts and fruit stones. At 10 or 11 months bite-size pieces can be introduced. Snacks such as raisins and oatcakes are suitable for slightly older children, but at around 9 months still stay with fruit for snacks. Fruit or fresh fruit with yoghurt can be used for desserts as children at this age don't ask for alternatives – and it is so good for them.

FOODS TO INTRODUCE:

Introduce foods one by one, being alert to any reactions.

Dairy Products: Yoghurt (live, 'bio', plain – can be sweetened with fresh fruit or small amount of molasses).

Grains: Corn, oats, rye, barley.

Vegetables: Jerusalem artichokes, bamboo shoots, Chinese leaf and pak choy, samphire, sweetcorn, rhubarb, cucumber with seeds.

Meat: Liver

Fruit: Fruits with small seeds such as raspberries, strawberries, blackberries, figs, kiwi fruit, lychees, rambutans, dates, grapes.

Fats: Butter (in moderation)

Menu 1

BREAKFAST
Oat porridge & banana
Breast or bottle

MID MORNING
Fruit or raisins
Breast or bottle

LUNCH
Vegetable sticks with Terrific
Tuna Sauce*
Fruit
Water

MID AFTERNOON
Fruit or rye crackers
Breast or bottle

TEA TIME
Peppy Barley Stew*
Fruit
Water

BED TIME
Breast or bottle

Menu 4

BREAKFAST
Breakfast rice*
Breast or bottle

MID MORNING
Fruit or rye crackers
Breast or bottle

LUNCH
Vegetable sticks with Saucy Avocado*
Oatcakes
Water

MID AFTERNOON
Fruit
Breast or bottle

TEA TIME
Asian sauté* with Salmon
Banana Soup*
Water

BED TIME
Breast or bottle

Menu 2

• • • • • • • • •

BREAKFAST
Sugar-free cornflakes with yoghurt
Breast or bottle

MID MORNING
Fruit or oatcake
Breast or bottle

LUNCH
Baked Beans & Mashed Parsnip
Fruit
Water

MID AFTERNOON
Fruit
Breast or bottle

TEA TIME
Brown rice with Mushroom &
Onion Sauce*
Fruit
Water

BED TIME
Breast or bottle

Menu 3

• • • • • • • • •

BREAKFAST
Rice & Barley Muesli *
Breast or bottle

MID MORNING
Fruit or crackers
Breast or bottle

LUNCH
Sunny Courgette Bake*
Fruit
Water

MID AFTERNOON
Fruit
Breast or bottle

TEA TIME
Spinach & Chickpeas* with Quinoa*
Fruit
Water

BED TIME
Breast or bottle

Menu 5

• • • • • • • • •

BREAKFAST
Scrambled Eggs with Rye Toast
Breast or bottle

MID MORNING
Raisins or rice crackers
Breast or bottle

LUNCH
Walnut & Celeriac Sticks*
Mashed Sweet Potato
Water

MID AFTERNOON
Fruit
Breast or bottle

TEA TIME
Vegetable Chilli* with Barley
Fruit
Water

BED TIME
Breast or bottle

Menu 6

• • • • • • • • •

BREAKFAST
Quinoa-Millet Porridge*
Breast or bottle

MID MORNING
Fruit or oatcakes
Breast or bottle

LUNCH
Brown rice & Courgette Sauce*
Fruit
Water

MID AFTERNOON
Fruit
Breast or bottle

TEA TIME
Coconut Fish Curry* & Lentils
Fruit
Water

BED TIME
Breast or bottle

SIMPLE STIR-FRY

Brown rice or Japanese buckwheat pasta is the perfect accompaniment.

4–6 SERVINGS

1 tsp sesame oil
1 tbsp olive oil
2 garlic cloves, finely chopped
1 medium onion, finely chopped
Filtered water or Herb Stock
   (see page 176)
250g/8oz mushrooms,
   trimmed and diced
2 medium carrots,
   trimmed and finely grated
180g/6oz broccoli, stalks
   peeled and diced, florets
   separated into their smallest
   parts
250g/8oz bean sprouts

FOR THE SAUCE:
2 tsp tamari
2 tsp water
1 tsp sake (optional)

Heat the oils in a wok and add the garlic, onion and 2 tbsp water or broth. Stir for about 1 minute. Add the mushrooms, stir, then cook until they have begun to wilt, about 1½ minutes. Add the carrots and stir, then add the broccoli with 2 more tbsp water or broth.
Cook, stirring constantly, for 4–5 minutes.
Add the bean sprouts, with more liquid if the vegetables are sticking, and cook, stirring constantly, for 1 minute. Transfer the vegetables to a warmed serving platter and return the wok to the heat.
Whisk the sauce ingredients together and pour them into the wok. Cook until the alcohol has evaporated, no more than 1 minute.
To serve, either pour the sauce over the vegetables or serve on the side. Purée before serving, if necessary.

LEMON BRUSSELS SPROUTS

This is blissfully simple and delicious. The olive oil–lemon dressing works equally well with other vegetables. Try it on green beans, courgettes or broccoli.

4 SMALL SERVINGS

250g/8oz Brussels sprouts, trimmed
   and cut into thin rounds
2 tsp extra-virgin olive oil
Grated zest from ½ lemon
1 tsp freshly squeezed lemon juice

Steam the sprouts over boiling water until they are tender crisp, about 5 minutes.
Whisk together the oil, lemon zest and lemon juice in a medium bowl. Add the hot sprouts, toss until they are coated in the dressing. Purée before serving, if necessary.

MUSHROOM & LEEK RISOTTO

4–6 SERVINGS

Shiitake mushrooms are the best in terms of taste and nutrients, but this is still delicious made with ordinary mushrooms.

1.25 litres/2 pints Herb Stock
    (see page 176)
2 tbsp extra-virgin olive oil
1 leek, well cleaned and diced
360g/12oz mushrooms, trimmed
    and diced
200g/7oz short-grain brown rice
2 tbsp unsalted butter (optional)
Sea salt to taste

Heat the broth so it is steaming, cover and keep hot.
Heat the oil and diced leek over medium heat in a saucepan, or in a frying pan that is at least 7.5cm/3in deep. Stir and cook until the leek begins to soften, about 2 minutes. Add the mushrooms, stir and cook until they darken and become tender, 3½ minutes. Add the rice and cook, stirring constantly, until it takes on a translucence, 2–4 minutes. Add enough of the broth to just cover the rice and cook, stirring constantly, until the rice has absorbed most of the liquid, about 15 minutes.
Add the remaining broth and bring to a boil. Reduce the heat so the liquid is simmering merrily, cover and cook until the rice is almost tender through, about 25 minutes.
Uncover the rice and stir until most, but not all, of the liquid has evaporated, 5–10 minutes. Stir in butter if desired, then remove the risotto from the heat. Let it sit, covered, until ready to serve. Leftovers can be frozen in ice-cube trays; add a little filtered water if necessary when defrosting.

WALNUT CELERIAC STICKS

4 SERVINGS

Walnut oil is rich in both omega-3 and omega-6 fats.

2 tbsp walnut oil
1 small handful fresh flat-leaf
    parsley leaves
1 small bunch fresh chives
1 medium celeriac
    (about 800g/26oz)

Place the oil in a large bowl. Finely chop the herbs and stir them into the oil.
Bring a large pan of water to a boil.
Peel the celeriac and cut it into 7.5cm × 5mm × 5mm/3 × ¼ × ¼ in sticks. Plunge the sticks into the boiling water and let it return to the boil. Cook until the celeriac is tender but still has plenty of texture and isn't mushy, about 8 minutes. Drain, then run cold water over it until it has cooled slightly.
Add the celeriac sticks to the dressing and toss until they are thoroughly coated. Serve immediately, or at room temperature. Purée before serving, if necessary.

GOLDEN GREEN WAGON WHEELS
• •

4–6 SERVINGS

2 tbsp ghee (see page 176) or
   extra-virgin olive oil
¼ tsp fennel seeds, crushed
1 small onion, finely chopped
1 garlic clove, finely chopped
500g/1lb okra
1 tsp turmeric
4 tbsp filtered water
1 tbsp unsweetened flaked
   coconut, or to taste

*If you've never tried okra, this recipe will make you, and your baby,
a convert.*

Heat the ghee and fennel seeds in a large, heavy-bottomed frying
pan over medium heat. Stir until the fennel seeds have browned
slightly and begin to pop, about 3 minutes. Add the onion and
garlic, stir, then cover and cook until the onion is translucent, 5–7
minutes. Check frequently to be sure the onion isn't sticking.
While the onion is cooking, trim the ends from the okra and cut
them into very thin rounds.
Add the okra to the onion mixture and stir. Add the turmeric and
water and stir again. Cook, stirring frequently, until the okra is
tender and golden, about 20 minutes. The okra will go through a
very sticky, elastic stage, but will emerge from that to be very
tender.
Remove the pan from the heat. Sprinkle over the coconut, cover
and let sit for up to 10 minutes before serving. Purée if necessary.

PEPPY BARLEY STEW
• •

4–6 SERVINGS

2 tbsp olive oil
1 medium onion, finely chopped
2 garlic cloves, finely chopped
1 medium carrot, finely chopped
250g/8oz mushrooms, finely
   chopped
100g/3½oz hulled barley
¼ tsp ground ginger
½ tsp ground cinnamon
½ tsp turmeric
¼ tsp ground nutmeg
Pinch ground cloves
¼tsp coriander seeds, ground
750ml/1¼ pints Herb Stock
   (see page 176)

*Barley is often overlooked, yet it is easy to prepare and children like
the texture. The exotic spices in this recipe lift this humble grain out
of the ordinary.*

Cook the oil, onion and garlic in a large, heavy-bottomed frying
pan over medium heat until the onions are translucent, about 5
minutes. Add the carrot, mushrooms and barley and cook,
stirring occasionally, just until the mushrooms begin to darken
and the barley starts to smell toasty, about 5 minutes.
Stir in the spices, then add the broth and stir. Bring to a boil.
Reduce the heat so the liquid is simmering merrily, cover and
cook until the barley is tender but not mushy, about 50 minutes.
Remove from the heat and serve. Purée if necessary.

VARIATION:
If you prefer, you can omit the barley and substitute buckwheat
groats. Cook the vegetables in the broth until they are tender,
about 30 minutes. In a separate pan, bring 500ml/16fl oz water to
a boil. Add 180g/6oz buckwheat, return to the boil and let cook
until it is nearly but not quite tender, about 5 minutes. Drain the
buckwheat and let it sit, tightly covered, until it is tender and
fluffy, about 10 minutes. Add it to the stew just before serving.

VEGETABLE CHILLI WITH QUINOA

4–6 SERVINGS

1 medium onion, finely chopped
2 garlic cloves, finely chopped
1 green pepper, cored, seeded and
    finely chopped
1 litre/1¾ pints filtered water
1 large can (800g/26oz) whole
    plum tomatoes
1 tbsp mild paprika
1 tbsp ground cumin
¼ tsp turmeric
½ tsp dried oregano
1 400g/14oz can kidney beans
    with no added sugar or salt,
    drained and rinsed
2 tbsp olive oil
100g/3½oz quinoa, rinsed

TO GARNISH (OPTIONAL):
1 small bunch fresh chives, finely
    chopped
1 orange, skin, pith and pips
    removed, segmented
Live plain yoghurt

This hearty chilli could be the start of a repertoire of vegetarian main meals to include regularly in your family's menu.

Heat the oil in a large stainless steel saucepan over medium-high heat. When it is hot but not smoking, add the onion, garlic and green pepper. Reduce the heat to medium and cook, stirring frequently, until the onion turns translucent, about 9 minutes. Add half the water, the tomatoes, spices and oregano. Mix well and bring to a boil. Cook for about 30 minutes, checking occasionally to be sure the mixture doesn't dry out. If it does, add a little more water to keep it soupy.

Add the remaining water and the beans, bring to a boil, and stir in the cooked quinoa (*see below*). Bring the mixture to a boil again, then reduce the heat so it is simmering merrily. Cook, partially covered, until the quinoa is tender and a little spiral on the outside of each grain has separated from the grain, about 15 minutes. Season to taste and serve, with the garnishes on the side if desired. The chilli is delicious immediately, although its flavour will mellow and deepen after 12 hours. Purée if necessary.

TO COOK THE QUINOA:
Place the quinoa and 500ml/16fl oz water in a small saucepan and bring to a boil over medium-high heat. Reduce the heat to medium, cover partially so the steam escapes, and cook at a slow boil for about 12 minutes. The grains should double in size, become translucent and crack open so the spiral germ is visible. Remove from the heat and let sit, covered, for about 1 minute. The quinoa is now ready to eat or to add to soups or stews.

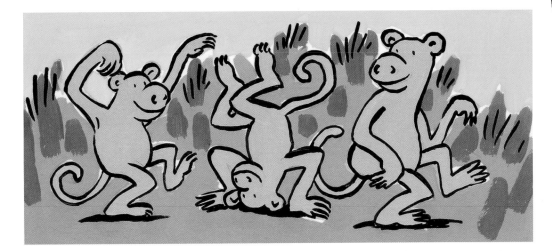

SUNNY COURGETTE BAKE

This will quickly become a family favourite. The crunchy topping can be added to all kinds of savoury or sweet dishes.

4–6 SERVINGS

500g/1lb courgettes, trimmed and
    finely grated
1 small onion, finely grated
Grated zest from ½ lemon
1 tsp freshly squeezed lemon juice

FOR THE TOPPING:
45g/1½oz rolled oats
4 tsp extra-virgin olive oil

Preheat the oven to 180°C/350°F/Gas 4.
In a medium bowl, toss together the courgettes, onion and lemon zest. Drizzle the lemon juice over all, toss again, then place in a small baking dish measuring about 28 × 18cm/11 × 7in.
Place the oats in a small bowl. Pour in the oil and toss the oats until the oil has soaked into them. Sprinkle the oats over the courgette mixture. Bake in the middle of the oven until the courgettes are tender and the topping is crisp, about 25 minutes.

AROMATIC DUCK BREASTS

This is simple to make and can also be finely ground in a food processor (add filtered water if necessary) for children as young as 6 months; be sure to remove the skin first.

4 SERVINGS

2 duck breasts
1 small garlic clove
¾ tsp five-spice powder

At least 1 hour (or up to 12 hours) before cooking the duck breasts, make 3 diagonal slits crosswise in the skin of the duck about 5mm/¼in deep. Evenly divide the garlic among the slits, pressing it down into them. Press equal amounts of the five-spice powder into the slits as well. Let the duck breasts sit at room temperature before cooking, to absorb the flavours.
Heat a cast-iron grill pan or frying pan over medium heat until hot but not smoking. Cook the duck breasts, skin-side down; until deep golden, about 10 minutes. Turn and continue cooking (10 additional minutes for medium, 6 minutes for rosy).
Remove and let sit for at least 10 and up to 20 minutes, to allow the juices to retreat back into the meat. To serve, either slice the duck breasts very, very thinly on the diagonal, or cut the meat into tiny, bite-sized pieces.

SPINACH AND CHICKPEAS
•••••••••••••••••••••••••••••••••••

Lentils can be used instead of chickpeas.

4 SERVINGS

1 tbsp ghee (see page 176) or olive
   oil
1 small onion, finely chopped
1 tbsp mild curry paste (preferably
   Patak's) or 1 tsp curry powder
180g/6oz cooked chickpeas
180g/6oz frozen spinach, or
   750g/1½lb fresh spinach,
   cooked
125ml/4fl oz unsweetened
   coconut milk

Melt the ghee in a medium saucepan over medium heat. Add the
onion, stir, then cook until it is translucent, about 5 minutes. Add
the curry paste or powder, stir, then add the chickpeas, spinach
and coconut milk. Bring to a boil, reduce the heat so the liquid is
simmering merrily, then cook for 10 minutes until the liquid has
reduced by about one-third. Remove from the heat, adjust the
seasoning and serve. Purée if necessary.

ASIAN SALMON BITES
•••••••••••••••••••••••••••••

Serve puréed for very small children.

4 SERVINGS

1 tsp sesame oil
1 tsp extra-virgin olive oil
1 garlic clove, finely chopped
500g/1lb salmon fillet, all bones
   and skin removed, cut into
   2.5cm/1in pieces
1 tbsp tamari
2 tbsp sake
4 tbsp filtered water

Heat the oils with the garlic in a medium frying pan over medium
heat until the garlic begins to turn translucent, about 2 minutes.
Add the salmon, stir, then add the remaining ingredients.
Stir until the salmon is cooked through and the liquids have
evaporated by half, 4–6 minutes. The result will be very moist
salmon, with a small amount of sauce.

MEDITERRANEAN MACKEREL FILLETS
•••••••••••••••••••••••••••

*Inexpensive and healthy, you will also be delighted that this is an easy
and delicious dish as well.*

4 SERVINGS

4 mackerel fillets, from fish that
   weighs about 500g/1lb, all
   bones removed
2 tsp extra-virgin olive oil
1 tsp dried oregano

Preheat the oven to its highest setting (about 230°C/450°F/Gas 9).
Brush the mackerel fillets with the oil and place in an ovenproof
baking dish. Cook for 5–8 minutes, or until cooked through.
Purée if necessary.

PEACH AND BANANA SMOOTHIE

MAKES ABOUT 1⅓ PINTS

500ml/16fl oz plain yoghurt
2 bananas, peeled and cut into
    small rounds
½ tsp vanilla extract
½ tsp ground cinnamon
1 medium peach, peeled, halved
    and stoned
1 tsp powdered blue-green algae
    (optional)

Blue-green algae is available from good health food shops and lends an interesting colour to this delicious drink. It is packed with trace minerals.

Place all the ingredients in a blender and process until smooth. This may be served as it is, diluted, or frozen in ice-cube trays or ice-lolly moulds and given to little ones to suck on.

AUTUMN NECTAR

MAKES ABOUT 500ML/ 16FL OZ

3 apples, cored and cut into
    chunks
2 large pears, cored and cut into
    chunks

Experiment with different apple varieties for more interesting flavours.

Place the fruit in a juicer and juice. Dilute before serving. This will keep 6–8 hours in the refrigerator.

SUNRISE DRINK

MAKES ABOUT 500ML/16FL OZ

125g/4oz fresh or frozen
    raspberries
1 mango, peeled, stoned and cut
    into 5cm/2in chunks
2 medium, slightly tart apples,
    cored and cut into chunks

Definitely not for children only.

Place all the fruits in a juicer and juice. Run the fruit through, alternating the apple with the mango, which has a tendency to slow down the machine.
Dilute before serving. This will keep 6–8 hours in the refrigerator.

FLAMING FRUIT JUICE

4 SERVINGS

This is a delicious way to sneak in some fresh carrots.

2 carrots, trimmed and cut into chunks
2 apples, cored and cut into eighths
125g/4oz mixed berries
90g/3oz grapes

Place all the ingredients in a juicer and juice. Dilute before serving. This will keep 6–8 hours in the refrigerator.

FRUIT NOG

4 SERVINGS

A filling snack and this treat delivers a host of nutrients as well.

250ml/8fl oz Autumn Nectar (see opposite)
1 banana, peeled
1 splash freshly squeezed lemon juice
Freshly ground nutmeg to taste (optional)

Place the nectar, banana and lemon juice in a blender and add nutmeg to taste if desired. Blend to a purée and dilute before serving. This will not keep.

Freshly Squeezed

THE FOLLOWING ARE GREAT FOR JUICES. IF USING A juicer, follow manufacturer's instructions for suitability. Some soft fruits, like bananas and blueberries, are better in a blender. Always serve diluted for small children.

FRUIT	Kiwi fruit	VEGETABLES
Apples	Mangoes	Beetroot
Apricots	Melons	Carrots
Bananas	Nectarines	Celery
Berries	Papayas	Cucumber
Cherries	Pears	Tomatoes
Citrus Fruit	Peaches	
Grapes	Pineapple	
	Plums	

12 - 15 MONTHS

CONTINUE WITH BREAST OR FORMULA MILK IF you wish, or begin to wean your child onto ordinary milk. If you have decided to avoid cow's milk, you can use goat or soya milk, or one of the other dairy substitutes (*see page 99*). Ensure your child is getting sufficient calcium and magnesium from a variety of foods including green leafy vegetables (*see page 69*). Meals can now consist of small cut-up chunks or finger foods.

FOODS TO INTRODUCE:

Introduce foods one by one, being alert to any reactions.

Protein Foods: Whole eggs, soya products, shellfish.

Vegetables: The deadly nightshade family: potatoes, tomatoes, aubergines, sweet peppers; olives (pits removed), salad leaves.

Fruit: Citrus fruit in small quantities avoiding oranges and grapefruit, passion fruit, pomegranates.

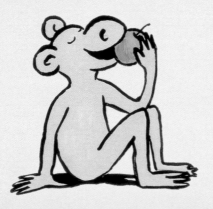

Menu 1

BREAKFAST
Sugar-free cornflakes
Fruit

MID MORNING
Raisins

LUNCH
Mushroom Tortilla*
Vegetable sticks

MID AFTERNOON
Fruit or rye crackers

TEA TIME
Bean & Garlic Stew*
Fruit

Menu 4

BREAKFAST
Scrambled eggs with
fresh herbs & fruit

MID MORNING
Raisins
or rice crackers

LUNCH
Chickpea Marbles*
Peas

MID AFTERNOON
Fruit

TEA TIME
Jacket potato with filling*
Fruit

Menu 2

• • • • • • • • • •

BREAKFAST
Porridge & fruit

MID MORNING
Rice cakes

LUNCH
Tofu Bites*
Steamed green vegetables

MID AFTERNOON
Fruit

TEA TIME
Coconut-Fish Curry*
& lentils
Pineapple Crisp*

Menu 3

• • • • • • • • • •

BREAKFAST
Rice & Barley Muesli* & fruit

MID MORNING
Fruit

LUNCH
Liver Pâté* on rye toast
Coleslaw*

MID AFTERNOON
Fruit

TEA TIME
East Indian Lamb Nuggets*
Sweetcorn
Fruit

Menu 5

• • • • • • • • • •

BREAKFAST
Quinoa-Millet Porridge*

MID MORNING
Fruit

LUNCH
Pitta fingers &
Vegetable sticks with dips*
Yoghurt

MID AFTERNOON
Fruit

TEA TIME
Corn Pasta with Tomato Sauce*
Fruit Salad*

Menu 6

• • • • • • • • • •

BREAKFAST
Baked beans
& brown rice

MID MORNING
Oatcakes

LUNCH
Potato & Cabbage Fritters*
Fruit

MID AFTERNOON
Fruit

TEA TIME
Roast Cod with Broccoli & Anchovy
Sauce* & Cannellini Beans

POLENTA WITH ROASTED VEGETABLES

Polenta (corn meal) is delicious, and easy to prepare. Any leftover pieces can be served with a pasta sauce (see Recipe Index).

4–6 SERVINGS

FOR THE POLENTA:
3 tbsp extra-virgin olive oil
250g/8oz coarse polenta
1 litre/1¾ pints filtered water

FOR THE VEGETABLES:
2 large red or green peppers (each about 200g/7oz), cored, seeded and cut into 5cm/2in chunks
2 large carrots (each about 125g/4oz), trimmed and cut into 5cm/2in lengths
3 small onions (each about 125g/4oz), cut into quarters
250g/8oz broccoli, stalks peeled, cut into bite-sized pieces
2 smallish aubergines (each about 200g/7oz), trimmed and cut into 5cm/ 2in chunks
10 garlic cloves (optional)
3 tbsp extra-virgin olive oil

Preheat the oven to 240°C/475°F/Gas 9.

Heat 1 tbsp of the oil with the polenta in a large, heavy-bottomed saucepan over medium heat and cook, stirring occasionally, until the polenta smells toasty, about 8 minutes. Add the water, stir, then bring to a boil. Cover and cook, stirring occasionally, until the polenta thickens and is tender, about 20 minutes. Check the polenta occasionally and add more water if necessary to keep it from sticking. Remove from the heat and pour the polenta onto a baking sheet lined with parchment paper. Make a 23 × 30cm/9 × 12in rectangle, smoothing it out as best you can. Let cool.

In a large bowl, toss all the vegetables with the oil, then transfer to a baking dish large enough to hold them in a single layer. Roast until the vegetables are tender but not overly darkened, about 40 minutes. After 30 minutes, check the vegetables and if the broccoli is getting too dark, simply remove it.

Preheat the grill. Brush the polenta lightly on each side with the remaining oil, then cut it into rectangular or diamond shapes. Grill until it is golden on one side, about 4 minutes. Turn and grill on the other side, another 4 minutes.

To serve, arrange the polenta on a serving platter and place the vegetables on top. Alternatively, serve the vegetables separately, in the dish in which they were roasted.

TOFU BITES

You may toss these into cooked brown rice, add them to soup, or simply serve as finger food.

4 APPETIZER SERVINGS

4 tsp tamari
1 tsp water
1 tsp sake
1 small garlic clove, finely chopped
1 thin disc fresh root ginger, peeled and finely chopped
125g/4oz tofu, cut into 1.25cm/½in squares
2 tsp vegetable oil
½ tsp sesame oil, or to taste

Place the tamari, water, sake, garlic and ginger in a shallow bowl. Mix, then add the tofu. Mix again, cover and marinate for at least 1 hour, or up to 8 hours.

Heat the vegetable oil in a non-stick frying pan over medium heat until it is hot. Add the tofu and its marinade, toss, then cook, stirring constantly, until the tofu cubes are golden and hot through, 4–5 minutes. Remove from the heat, drizzle with sesame oil to taste and serve.

Jacket potato fillings

JACKET POTATOES ARE PARTICULARLY valuable because, cooked whole, they retain most of their nutrients. They are a good source of complex carbohydrates and the skin, along with the few millimetres beneath the skin, contains fibre, vitamin C and some B vitamins including folic acid, and iron. If you cook potatoes in any way other than baking them, such as steaming or boiling, it is best to keep their skins on and peel them, if you must, after they are cooked. Discard any potatoes that have a green tinge, or cut that bit out, as it contains solanine which is toxic.

As potatoes are a member of the deadly nightshade family they contain some compounds that may be troublesome to very small children and so ideally should not be introduced until the age of 12 months. Don't let this put you off once your child is old enough, as the majority of people can tolerate this delicious and satisfying alkaline food. For younger children you could use alternative starchy bases such as sweet potato (not the same family), yam, swede or brown rice.

For fillings, it is quite handy to keep some leftovers of a meal, for example ratatouille, and freeze it as a quick topping to add to a potato for an almost instant meal. Here are some suggested toppings. I'm sure you can dream up more:

VEGETARIAN:
Tomato, onion and olive cooked in a little wine (cooking burns off the alcohol)
Guacomole
Ratatouille
Hummus*
Mild vegetable curry in coconut sauce
Mushrooms cooked with olive oil, garlic, lemon and a little wine
Salsa
Coleslaw*
Baked beans
Sliced baby leeks, cooked with olive oil and a little wine
No-salt or sugar tinned beans, cooked with diced onions, olive oil and a pinch of curry powder or paste
Vegetable chilli*
Spinach with chickpeas*
Roasted vegetables*
Bean and garlic stew*
Saucy Avocado* & cooked kidney beans

DAIRY:
Yoghurt and chives
Tzatziki (Greek yoghurt with cucumber and mint)
Cottage cheese, avocado and chopped spring onions
Grilled goat's cheese with red peppers
Finely chopped spinach and feta cheese
Grated goat's Cheddar and broccoli
Creamed sweetcorn, diced red peppers and chives

FISH AND MEAT:
Tuna with diced peppers and yoghurt-curry sauce*
Tuna dip*
Diced chicken and vegetables with saucy avocado*
Sardines in tomato sauce
Salmon, fresh or tinned, with peas & vinaigrette
Minced lamb with Courgette Sauce*

EAST INDIAN LAMB NUGGETS

These are a perfect finger food.

4 GENEROUS SERVINGS

FOR THE LAMB NUGGETS:
875g/1¾lb minced lamb
½ tsp ground coriander
¾ tsp ground cumin
2 garlic cloves, finely chopped
½ tsp ground ginger
1 shallot, finely chopped
1 tbsp freshly squeezed lemon juice

TO COOK THE LAMB NUGGETS:
2 tbsp extra-virgin olive oil
½ tsp ground cinnamon
4 cardamom pods
¼ tsp ground cloves
¼ tsp ground coriander
½ tsp turmeric
½ tsp paprika
1 medium onion, finely chopped
2 tbsp water
Live plain yoghurt and diced
*   cucumber, to garnish (optional)*

To make the lamb nuggets, mix all the ingredients together and shape into small patties.

To cook, heat the oil and spices in a heavy frying pan over medium heat until the oil begins to sizzle. Add the lamb nuggets (which can be slightly crowded but must be in one layer in the pan) and cook until they are golden all over and nearly cooked through, 6–8 minutes. Remove them from the pan and set aside. Add the onion and water to the pan and stir and scrape to get up all the browned bits from the bottom of the pan. Cook, stirring frequently, until the onion is softened and tender, about 20 minutes. You may want to add more water – the onion shouldn't be dry, nor should it stick to the bottom of the pan. Return the lamb nuggets and their cooking juices to the pan, cover and heat through.

To serve, transfer the nuggets, onion and any cooking juices to a serving platter or bowl and serve immediately, with the garnishes on the side if desired.

CHICKPEA MARBLES

These tasty little bites are best warm, not hot or cold. Hot, they burn little fingers; cold they lose their charm.

4–6 SERVINGS

360g/12oz cooked chickpeas
1 tbsp mild curry paste
1 tsp live yoghurt
1 large egg
750ml/1¼ pints mild
*   vegetable oil*

Place the chickpeas in a food processor and blend until they are finely ground. Add the remaining ingredients and blend until everything is thoroughly mixed.

Heat the oil in a medium, heavy-bottomed saucepan and heat over medium-high heat until it is hot but not smoking.

Form marble-sized balls with the chickpea mixture. Fry them in small batches (so they do not crowd the pan) until they are golden, 3–4 minutes. Transfer to a plate lined with paper towels to drain. Serve when they are cool enough to handle.

POTATO AND CABBAGE FRITTERS

4 SERVINGS

Another healthy and delicious finger-food offering.

500g/1lb starchy potatoes, peeled and cut into chunks
125g/4oz cabbage, diced
4tbsp flat-leafed parsley leaves
1 small bunch fresh chives
1–2 tbsp extra-virgin olive oil
Yoghurt Curry Dressing (see page 177), to serve (optional)

Place the potatoes and cabbage in a steamer over boiling water, keeping them separate. Cover and steam until they are both tender, 20 minutes. Remove the vegetables from the steamer. Mash the potatoes with a fork, add the cabbage and mix until blended, then stir in the parsley and chives. Form the mixture into 8 patties.

Preheat the oven to 240°C/475°F/Gas 9.

Place 1 tbsp of the oil in a cast-iron, ovenproof frying pan and place in the oven to heat until the oil is hot but not smoking. Place the patties in the pan, return to the oven and bake until they are golden on one side, about 5 minutes. Flip the patties over, add the additional oil if necessary, then continue baking until they are golden on the other side, about 5 minutes. Serve with yoghurt dressing on the side, if desired.

Easy Liver pâté

LIVER IS PACKED WITH NUTRIENTS SO IT IS A good idea to offer it to your child from the age of nine months, but organic is best *(see page 81)*. Because of the high vitamin A content, it is best to offer only occasionally, about once every other week is ideal.

If you have a source of organic chicken, then chances are good that you can get organic chicken livers, which can be used for a delicious 'quickie' pâté. To prepare, cut the liver into small pieces removing any strings and fibrous parts. Finely chop half of one small onion. Heat about 1 tbsp extra-virgin olive oil in a small frying pan, add the onion and liver and cook, stiring often, until cooked through, 5–8 minutes. Stir in 2 tbsp dry sherry (or apple juice) and a small handful of chopped raisins. Cook until the liquid has evaporated. Serve as is, spread on toasted bread or rye crackers. The mixture can be puréed for small children. This will keep for 2–3 days, covered, in the refrigerator.

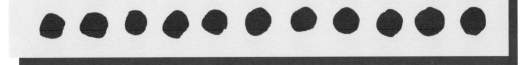

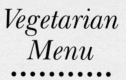

IDEAS FOR BIRTHDAY PARTIES

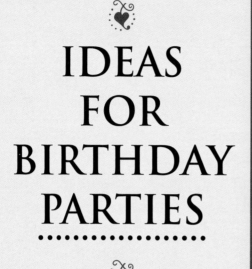

Y OUR CHILD'S FIRST BIRTHDAY PARTY IS such fun, but choosing the healthy options can be a bit of a nuisance – unless you are armed with ideas. Here are some healthy birthday party menu suggestions, suitable for children 12 months and over. Your child and his friends will love it. For the cake, try the Apple Cake recipe on page 157 and be sure to allow enough for the adults – it's delicious.

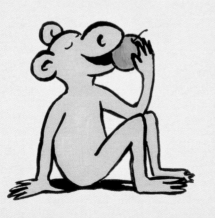

Vegetarian Menu

Chickpea Marbles*

Bite-size oven-roasted potato cubes

Carrot & Cucumber sticks with Yoghurt-Curry Sauce*

Corn chips

Cherry tomato quarters

Apple wedges

Raisins

Simple Menu 2

East Indian Lamb Nuggets*

Sweetcorn Kernels & Peas

Corn Pasta Shapes with Olive Oil & Grated Parmesan

Vegetable sticks with Saucy Avocado*

Popcorn

Melon Balls

Sophisticated Menu

· · · · · · · ·

Smoked mackerel pâté on oatcakes

Potato & Cabbage Fritters*

Steamed broccoli florets

Carrot & Cucmber sticks with
Terrific Tuna Sauce*

Avocado Chunks

Blueberries & Pear Slices

Dried cherries

Oriental Menu

· · · · · · · ·

Tofu bites*

Asian salmon*

Sliced, stir-fried mushrooms
& sugar snap peas
(remove any strings)

Cucumber sticks & rice cakes

Flavoured Japanese rice crackers
(be sure these do not contain whole
nuts because they are a choking
hazard)

Papaya & Banana Chunks

Italian Menu

· · · · · · · ·

Pasta Shapes with Tomato Sauce*

Mini Polenta Pizzas*

Meatballs

Vegetable Sticks
with Terrific Tuna Sauce*

Oven-roasted courgette fingers

Assorted stoned olives

Red & Green Grapes
(cut in half & pips removed)

Other good party foods

· · · · · · · · · · · ·

Fish cakes

Vegetarian Sausages & Peas

Falafel

Oatcakes with
cashew nut butter
& 100% fruit jam

Salmon Dumplings*

Oven-roasted root vegetable chunks

Rye toast squares with spreads

Sugar-free corn flakes

Fresh fruit juices & smoothies*

SAUTÉED APPLES

4 SERVINGS

1 tbsp unsalted butter
2 medium apples, cored, peeled
    and cut into thin slices
Ground cinnamon and nutmeg,
    to serve (optional)

This is simple and delicious.

Melt the butter in a non-stick frying pan and add the apple slices. Cook, stirring and shaking the pan constantly, until the apples are golden and soft, about 7 minutes. Remove from the heat, dust with the spices if desired, and serve.

PINEAPPLE CRISP

4–6 SERVINGS

500g/1lb fresh pineapple rings
5 tbsp pineapple or apple juice
1 tbsp unsalted butter
2 tbsp blackstrap molasses
1 tbsp freshly squeezed lemon juice
120g/4oz rolled oats
½ tsp freshly grated nutmeg
Plain yoghurt, to serve (optional)

Pudding has never tasted so good, with a delightful contrast of textures.

Preheat the oven to 190°C/375°F/Gas 5.
Place the pineapple rings in a baking dish large enough to hold them in a single layer. Pour the juice over them.
In a small saucepan, melt together the butter and molasses. Place the oats in a medium bowl, pour the butter and molasses over them, then toss until all the ingredients are combined.
Sprinkle the nutmeg evenly over the pineapple, then sprinkle the oat mixture evenly on top, making sure the pineapple is covered with topping and slightly mounded with it in the middle.
Bake in the middle of the oven until the topping is crisp, about 35–40 minutes.
Remove from the oven and let cool for about 10 minutes before serving.
To serve, using a spatula or pie server, place 1–2 pineapple rings on individual dessert plates, with yoghurt if desired.

APPLE CAKE
• • • • • • • • • • • • • •

MAKES TWO 23CM/9IN CAKES

2 medium apples, grated
135g/4½oz raisins
185ml/6fl oz mild honey
½ tsp ground cinnamon
½ tsp ground allspice
½ tsp ground ginger
½ tsp freshly grated nutmeg
⅛ tsp ground cloves
2 tbsp unsalted butter
375ml/12fl oz water
290g/9½oz fine cornmeal
1 tsp bicarbonate of soda
45g/1½oz top-quality, organic,
   bittersweet or milk chocolate

This cake is delectably spicy, and surprisingly light. It can also be made successfully with the same quantity of wholewheat flour, instead of the cornmeal.

Preheat the oven to 150°C/300°F/Gas 2. Butter and lightly flour two 23cm/9in cake tins.
Place the apples, raisins, honey, spices and butter in a medium saucepan. Stir in the water and bring to a boil over medium heat. Cover and cook until the apples are soft, 10 minutes. Remove from the heat and let cool.
Combine the cornmeal and bicarbonate of soda in a large bowl. Stir in the liquid ingredients and mix until just combined. Pour half the mixture into each of the prepared tins and bake until the cakes are golden and spring back when touched, 35–40 minutes. Remove the cakes from the oven and place on wire racks. Grate equal amounts of chocolate over each cake, then let the cakes cool before removing them from the tins.
To serve, you may either stack the layers, or serve them individually.

BANANA SOUP
• • • • • • • • • • • • • •

4–6 SERVINGS

3 good-sized bananas
4 cubes dried apricot purée
   (see page 131)
2–3 tsp freshly squeezed lemon
   juice
70g/2½oz berries (optional)
Unsweetened flaked coconut, to
   serve (optional)

This dessert is wonderfully sinful, and yet it is 100% healthy!

Peel the bananas and place the flesh in a food processor with the apricot purée and lemon juice. Purée until light and foamy.
Add the berries if desired, purée, then transfer to a serving dish. Chill, covered, for up to 1 hour.
To serve, dust with coconut if desired.

15 - 24 MONTHS

ONCE YOU HAVE ADDED IN THE FOODS BELOW, your child will be fully weaned onto a wide variety of foods and you can feed him any meals that are being eaten by the whole family (keeping salt and sugar to a minimum).

FOODS TO INTRODUCE:

Introduce foods one by one, being alert to any reactions.

Fruit: Oranges and Grapefruit

Grains: Wheat in rotation with other grains – it is wise not to become too dependent on wheat.

Dairy products: Milk and cheese – it is wise to keep the emphasis on goat's and sheep's milk cheese and to keep cow's milk to a sensible minimum.

Seeds: Ground sunflower, pumpkin, sesame, linseeds, pine kernels or sprouted seeds. These can be introduced earlier, at around 9 months (finely ground) if you are not concerned about having a child with potential allergies. They are a very good source of minerals, fibre and essential fats.

Nuts: Introduce last of all if concerned about allergies, otherwise introduce earlier as they are an excellent source of nutrients; almonds, chestnuts, walnuts, pistachios, brazils, hazelnuts, cashews, pecan and others. See page 65 for more information on peanuts.

Menu 1

BREAKFAST
Wholewheat toast with
100% fruit spread
Cottage cheese

MID MORNING
Raisins
Milk

LUNCH
Chicken Nibbles*
Thinly sliced celery & carrots

MID AFTERNOON
Fruit or rye crackers

TEA TIME
Mediterranean Rice*
Fruit

Menu 4

BREAKFAST
Porridge & fruit

MID MORNING
Raisins

LUNCH
Pasta with
Walnut Pesto*
Fruit

MID AFTERNOON
Fruit

TEA TIME
Baked Chicken with
Golden Green Wagon Wheels*
Apple Cake*

Menu 2
• • • • • • • • • •

BREAKFAST
Sugar-free cornflakes & fruit

MID MORNING
Fruit

LUNCH
Pitta fingers with Hummus*
& Tabbouleh*
Avocado slices

MID AFTERNOON
Fruit

TEA TIME
Grilled fresh sardines
& steamed vegetables

Menu 3
• • • • • • • • • •

BREAKFAST
Baked beans
& mushrooms

MID MORNING
Mini rice cakes

LUNCH
Potato Gratin*
Steamed carrots

MID AFTERNOON
Fruit
Date Oat Wedges*

TEA TIME
Polenta & Roasted Vegetables*

Menu 5
• • • • • • • • • •

BREAKFAST
Quinoa-Millet Porridge*,
ground seeds & yoghurt

MID MORNING
Raisins

LUNCH
Brown rice with Broccoli
& Anchovy Sauce*
Fruit

MID AFTERNOON
Fruit or crackers

TEA TIME
Mini-pizza*
Fruit Salad*

Menu 6
• • • • • • • • • •

BREAKFAST
Quinoa* porridge & fruit

MID MORNING
Rice cakes

LUNCH
Fish Fingers* & Coleslaw*
Indian Pudding*

MID AFTERNOON
Fruit

TEA TIME
Baked Sweet Potato
& Steamed Broccoli
Fruit or yoghurt

POTATO, PEAS, PASTA

4 SERVINGS

1 large potato (270g/9oz), peeled and cut into 5mm/¼in squares
30g/1oz fresh or frozen peas
250g/8oz cooked pasta
1 tbsp extra-virgin olive oil
Fresh sage, thyme or parsley, to garnish (optional)

Use pasta shells with this sauce so that the potatoes and peas can hide inside them.

Steam the potatoes over boiling water until they are almost tender, about 10 minutes. Add the peas and steam until they are tender and hot through, about 5 minutes for fresh peas, 7–8 minutes for frozen.
In a medium bowl, toss all the ingredients together. Garnish with the fresh herbs if desired.

GOLDEN CAULIFLOWER PASTA SAUCE

4–6 SERVINGS

360g/12oz cauliflower florets, finely chopped
1 shallot, finely chopped
¼ tsp turmeric
250ml/8fl oz filtered water
1 tbsp extra-virgin olive oil
360g/12oz warm cooked pasta

This is a delicious and easy way to serve cauliflower.

Place the cauliflower, shallot, turmeric and water in a non-stick frying pan over medium heat. Stir and bring to a boil. Cook, stirring occasionally, until the cauliflower is tender and the water has evaporated, 10–15 minutes.
Add the oil, stir, and continue to cook until the cauliflower is tender through and just beginning to turn slightly golden at the edges, 4–5 minutes.
Transfer the cauliflower to a large bowl, add the pasta and toss until well blended. Serve.

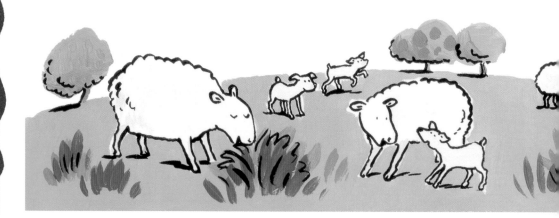

COURGETTE PASTA SAUCE

4–6 SERVINGS

Pasta shells or macaroni turn this sauce into perfect finger food.

1 garlic clove, finely chopped
250ml/8fl oz filtered water
1 courgette, weighing about
    250g/8oz, trimmed and diced
1 tsp fresh thyme leaves
1 tbsp olive oil
250g/8oz warm cooked pasta
Grated Parmesan cheese, to serve
    (optional)

Place the garlic and 2 tbsp of the water in a non-stick frying pan over medium heat, making sure the garlic is covered with the water. Cook until the water has evaporated. Add the courgette, the remaining water and the thyme and cook, stirring occasionally, until the water has evaporated and the courgette is tender, about 15 minutes. Remove from the heat and stir in the olive oil, then toss with the warm pasta. Serve with Parmesan cheese if desired.

MUSHROOM & ONION SAUCE

4–6 SERVINGS

Serve this sauce with wagon wheel pasta.

1 large onion, diced
250ml/8fl oz filtered water
250g/8oz mushrooms, trimmed,
    wiped clean and diced
1 dried bay leaf
360g/12oz warm cooked pasta
2–4tsp extra-virgin olive oil

Place the onion and half the water in a non-stick frying pan over medium heat. Bring the water to a boil and cook until it has almost all evaporated, 7–10 minutes.
Add the mushrooms, the remaining water and the bay leaf. Stir and bring to a boil, then cover and cook until the mushrooms and onions are soft, about 15 minutes.
Uncover the pan and continue cooking, stirring occasionally, until the liquid has almost all evaporated. Place the mushroom and onion sauce in a medium bowl with the pasta. Drizzle with as much oil as you like and toss the ingredients until they are thoroughly blended. Serve.

TOMATO SAUCE
●●●●●●●●●●●●●●●●●●●●●●●

Tomatoes are the best source of lycopene, one of the carotenoids that are most helpful in protecting against cancer.

1kg/2lb tomatoes, cored, peeled and cut horizontally in half, or 800g/26oz can whole plum tomatoes
1 small onion, diced
1 garlic clove, finely chopped
1 small handful fresh basil leaves
1½ tbsp extra-virgin olive oil (optional)

Place the tomatoes, onion and garlic in a medium casserole over medium heat and bring to a boil. Reduce the heat so the mixture is bubbling gently and cook until the tomatoes have softened but not really lost their shape, about 15 minutes.

Coarsely chop the basil and stir it into the sauce. Continue to cook until the tomatoes are very soft but not mushy, an additional 15 minutes. They should still be bright in colour.

Remove from the heat, stir in the olive oil if desired, and either use immediately over pasta, or freeze.

WONDERFUL WALNUT PESTO
●●●●●●●●●●●●●●●●●●●●●

When tossing this sauce with cooked pasta, you may need to moisten it with a little of the cooking water from the pasta.

4–6 SERVINGS

1 garlic clove
30g/1oz chunk Parmesan cheese, grated
45g/1½oz walnuts
100g/3½oz fresh basil
4 tbsp extra-virgin olive oil

Place the garlic, cheese and walnuts in a mortar and pestle (or a food processor) and grind or process until they are very finely chopped and well-combined. Add the basil and grind or process until it is very finely chopped, then add the oil in a fine stream, mixing or processing all the while so it combines well with the other ingredients.

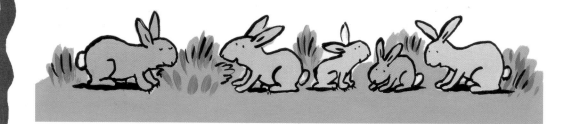

BROCCOLI AND ANCHOVY PASTA SAUCE

4 SERVINGS

This sauce is best with pasta shapes.

135g/4½oz broccoli florets
2 anchovy fillets
3 tbsp extra-virgin olive oil
Grated zest from ½ lemon
    (optional)

Steam the broccoli over boiling water until it is tender, about 8 minutes. Remove from the heat.
Sauté the anchovies in the oil, stirring and breaking them up. Add the broccoli and cook, stirring and breaking up the florets until they are almost a rough purée and hot through, 3–4 minutes. Add the lemon zest if desired, remove from the heat and toss with the cooked pasta.
If the sauce is not moist enough, add a little pasta cooking water to moisten it.

Pasta Varieties

WHEN AIMING TO REDUCE OR CUT OUT wheat from your child's diet, one of the easiest ways to offer alternatives is to choose from the wide range of pastas that can be found instead of ordinary durum wheat pasta.

Wheat is very high in gluten, which is a sticky protein that fills with air when cooked, (this is why it is ideal for bread-baking). It also ensures that pasta is light, another attribute that makes it popular. But it is this very gluten that makes it such a problem with allergies.

If you must use wheat pasta, it is always a better option to use the wholewheat brown pasta that is readily available in a variety of shapes and sizes. Of course occasional use of the fresh, flavoured pastas will do no harm in moderation – just remember that they are refined and therefore not nutritionally complete. If organic flour is used then so much the better.

Most good health food shops will offer alternative pastas in many shapes and some may be coloured with spinach or tomato for variety. They are available made from corn, rice, millet and rye. Be warned, however, they do not cook quite like the pasta that you may be used to. They do not take much longer to cook, but they do tend to be a bit 'heavier'. In fact you may need to use less to satisfy a hungry appetite. Japanese 'Udon' noodles are made from buckwheat. Follow cooking instructions on the packet as they cook a little differently to normal pasta. Chinese rice noodles are another option, though they are refined. These are both delicious with a simple dressing of soya sauce and a little sesame oil.

Explore all the options, and remember the greater the variety of ingredients you use, the greater the number of nutrients you offer your child.

Hummus
● ● ● ● ● ● ● ● ● ● ●

6–10 servings

475g/15oz dried chickpeas, sprouted and cooked (see below)
2 large garlic cloves
3–4 tbsp sesame tahini
4–6 tbsp freshly squeezed lemon juice
3 tbsp extra-virgin olive oil
Warm filtered water (if necessary)

This is my all-time favourite fast food. It works well with pitta bread, vegetable sticks or just a spoon and is great as a topping for baked potatoes.

Place the chickpeas, garlic and 3 tbsp tahini in the bowl of a food processor and process 2 or 3 times. With the food processor running, add 4 tbsp lemon juice and 2 tbsp olive oil, and continue processing until you have a smooth, soft purée. If the purée is very, very thick, leave the food processor running and add enough warm water to make a purée to the consistency you desire. Taste and adjust the seasoning, adding more tahini and lemon juice if desired.

Transfer to a serving bowl and flatten the hummus except for a slight mound in the middle. Using your finger, trace indentations away from the middle to the outer edge of the bowl. Pour the remaining olive oil in the middle of the hummus and it will run down the indentations, creating a nice pattern. Serve immediately.

To sprout the chickpeas
Place them in a bowl, cover with warm water and let sit overnight. Drain off the water, rinse the beans and return them to their bowl. Add enough water to not quite cover them (but so they are moist). Rinse and repeat several times a day for about 3 days, until you see sprouts form. They are now ready to use in the recipe.

Gazpacho Salad
● ●

4 servings

2 medium tomatoes, peeled, cored and diced
½ green pepper, cored, seeded and diced
½ avocado, peeled, stoned and diced
1 small cucumber, or 1 × 7.5cm/3in long chunk of cucumber, peeled and diced
1tsp freshly squeezed lemon juice
1 small handful fresh basil leaves
1–2tbsp extra-virgin olive oil
90 –125g/3–4oz sheep's milk feta cheese

If your child is not fond of salads, then spread this on a round of wholewheat pitta bread and place under a hot grill until the cheese just melts – gazpacho pizza will go down very well.

Combine the vegetables in a medium bowl. Add the lemon juice and toss. If the basil leaves are very small, leave them whole, otherwise tear them into bite-sized pieces. Add the basil to the salad, toss thoroughly, then transfer to a shallow bowl. Drizzle with 1tbsp olive oil.

Crumble the amount of feta cheese you like over the salad, then drizzle with another 1tbsp olive oil and garnish with additional basil leaves, if desired.

CREAMY COLESLAW

4 SERVINGS

6 tbsp plain yoghurt
2 tbsp pineapple juice
½ small white (750g/1½lb)
  cabbage, cored and finely
  chopped

TO GARNISH:
30g/1oz sunflower seeds
¼–½ tsp ground cumin
1 small bunch fresh chives
  (optional)

This recipe is also good with red cabbage, or use half the weight of cabbage and the other half of grated carrot.

In a large bowl, whisk together the yoghurt and pineapple juice. Add the cabbage, toss until it is thoroughly coated with the dressing, then cover and refrigerate for at least 20 minutes.
Place the sunflower seeds in a small, heavy-bottomed frying pan over medium heat. Cook, stirring frequently, until they are evenly golden, about 4 minutes. Remove from the heat and let cool.
In a food processor, grind the seeds with cumin to taste until they are finely chopped. Finely chop the chives, if using.
Either sprinkle the sunflower seeds and chives on top of the salad just before serving, or serve the salad plain, with the garnishes alongside.

TABBOULEH

4–6 SERVINGS

125g/4oz bulgur
500ml/16fl oz boiling filtered
  water
250g/8oz tomatoes, cored and
  diced
125g/4oz cucumber, peeled and
  diced
20g/¾ oz flat-leaf parsley leaves
4 tbsp chopped fresh mint
3 tbsp freshly squeezed lemon
  juice, or to taste
3 tbsp extra-virgin olive oil
¼ tsp ground cumin (optional)

Even children who do not like salads eat this with relish.

Place the bulgur in a medium bowl, cover with the boiling water and let sit for 1 hour.
Drain the bulgur thoroughly and return it to the bowl. Add the remaining ingredients and toss thoroughly. Let sit for 1 hour or overnight before serving.

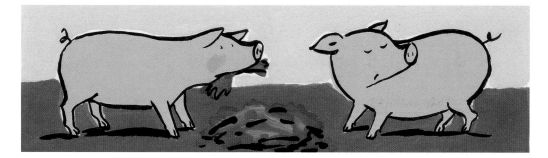

WONDER FOODS 15 - 24 MONTHS

THIS MEAL PLANNER WILL GIVE YOU a good idea of how easy it is to incorporate the advice given on pages 76–79. All Wonder Food ingredients appear in *italics*. Many of these menus can also be adapted for younger age groups. With the exception of game, most of the Wonder Foods offer economical as well as nutritious menu possibilities.

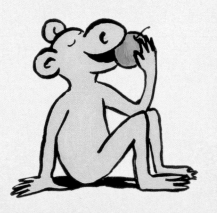

Day 1

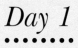

BREAKFAST
Oat porridge
& grated *apple*

SNACK
Raisins

LUNCH
Tinned *mackerel* on rye toast
Grapes

SNACK
Fruit

TEA TIME
Venison Stew*
& Steamed Vegetables
Fruit

Day 4

BREAKFAST
Baked beans & *mushrooms*
*Cantaloupe**

SNACK
*Oat*cakes

LUNCH
Onion soup
Wholewheat toast
with *sunflower seed* spread

SNACK
Fruit

TEA TIME
Asian *Salmon* Bites*
Brown rice with *seaweed* flakes

Day 2

BREAKFAST
Rice & Barley Muesli*

SNACK
Yoghurt

LUNCH
Pitta fingers & vegetable sticks
with *Hummus**
*Apricots**

SNACK
Fruit

TEA TIME
Tuna with Twenty *Garlic* Cloves*
Lentils
Fruit

Day 3

BREAKFAST
Scrambled eggs
& smoked *salmon* trimmings
Rye toast
Fruit

SNACK
Date *Oat* Wedges*

LUNCH
Corn pasta with *Broccoli*
& Anchovy Sauce*
Fruit

SNACK
Fruit

TEA TIME
Stir-fried tofu with *carrots,
cabbage* & *shiitake mushrooms*
Brown rice
*Papaya**

Day 5

BREAKFAST
Breakfast rice with *ground seeds*
Pineapple

SNACK
Raisins

LUNCH
Mediterranean *Mackerel**
Lemon *Brussels Sprouts**

SNACK
Fruit

TEA TIME
Baked *Pumpkin* with Potato Gratin*
Apple slices*

Day 6

BREAKFAST
Quinoa-Millet Porridge*
Papaya

SNACK
Yoghurt & *molasses*

LUNCH
Potato & *Cabbage* Fritters*
Fruit

SNACK
Fruit

TEA TIME
Pheasant with *Apricots**
Steamed *Broccoli*
Brown rice

COCONUT FISH CURRY

You can use any other meaty fish instead of the tuna suggested here, and fresh or frozen peas substitute well for the broccoli.

4 SERVINGS

250g/8oz fresh tuna, skin and
   bones removed
60g/2oz broccoli, stalks peeled and
   cut into tiny cubes, florets cut
   into small pieces
1 small potato (90g/3oz), cut into
   1.25cm/ ½in cubes
1 tbsp extra-virgin olive oil
1 small onion, finely chopped
2–3 tsp mild curry paste
   (preferably Patak's) or 1 tsp
   curry powder
125ml/4fl oz unsweetened coconut
   milk
1 small handful fresh coriander
   leaves, to garnish (optional)

Rinse the fish and pat it dry. Cut it into 1.25cm/½in cubes and refrigerate until just before using.

Steam the broccoli and potato, covered, over boiling water until almost tender, 8–10 minutes. Remove and set aside.

Heat the oil and onion together and cook until the onion is nearly tender, about 10 minutes. Add the curry paste or powder, stir, then add the broccoli and potatoes.

Stir in the coconut milk and bring to a boil. Add the fish and adjust the heat so the coconut milk is simmering, then cook until the fish is opaque through, 5–8 minutes.

Serve over rice or by itself, with coriander as a garnish if desired. Mash with a fork if necessary.

PHEASANT WITH APRICOTS

This is a splurge but game is one of the Wonder Foods (see page 76). Be sure to remove any lead shot before serving.

4–6 SERVINGS

1.25–1.5kg/2½–3lb pheasant,
   cleaned
1 bay leaf
250g/8oz dried apricots
250g/8oz small onions, or
   medium onions cut into
   quarters
1–2 tbsp extra-virgin olive oil
125–185ml/4–6fl oz filtered
   water or Herb Stock (see page
   176)

Preheat the oven to 230°C/450°F/Gas 8.

Rinse the body cavity of the pheasant and place the bay leaf inside. Truss the bird if desired, then place in a flameproof baking dish large enough to hold it with room to spare. Scatter the apricots and onions around the pheasant, drizzle oil over everything, then pour 125ml/4fl oz water or broth over the apricots and onions.

Bake in the middle of the oven until the pheasant is cooked through, about 55 minutes (the leg bones should move freely when wiggled, and the juices that run from the leg joints should run clear when they are pricked with a skewer). If the apricots and onions are drying out and becoming too dark, drizzle additional water over them, and drape a piece of aluminium foil loosely over all.

Remove the dish from the oven, then remove the pheasant from the dish and turn it on its breast. Let it sit for at least 10 minutes (but preferably 20 minutes) before carving.

Just before serving, reheat the apricots and onions on top of the stove, adding additional water or broth if necessary so they are slightly moist. Stir them as they reheat, scraping up all the brown bits from the bottom of the dish. Serve immediately.

VENISON STEW
· · · · · · · · · · · · · · · · · · ·

4–6 SERVINGS

1 tbsp extra-virgin olive oil
750g/1½lb venison, cut into
    5cm/2in squares
1 small fennel bulb, trimmed and
    diced
12 pearl or spring onions,
    trimmed and left whole
3 carrots, trimmed and diced
250g/8oz mushrooms, trimmed,
    brushed clean and cut into
    quarters
1 bay leaf
1 small bunch fresh thyme or ½ tsp
    dried
2 × 5cm/2in strips orange zest
1 large sweet potato, peeled and
    cut into 1.25cm/½in squares

*This stew improves with age. If you refrigerate it overnight, the next
day you can skim off any fat that has risen to the top for a fat-free dish.
Beef can be used instead of venison.*

Heat the oil in a large, flameproof casserole or saucepan over
medium heat. Add the meat and brown it on all sides. Add the
fennel, onions, and carrots and cook, stirring, until the onions are
beginning to turn translucent. Add the mushrooms and stir, then
cover and cook, stirring occasionally, until the mushrooms have
begun to wilt and any liquid they give up is nearly absorbed back
into the vegetables, 5–8 minutes.

Cover the meat with hot water, add the herbs and orange zest and
bring to a boil. Reduce the heat so the liquid is simmering gently
and cook, partially covered, until the meat is tender, about 2
hours. Check occasionally to be sure the level of the liquid just
covers the meat, and add additional hot water if necessary.

Add the sweet potato and stir, then cover and cook until the
pieces of potato are tender through, about 15 minutes. Remove
from the heat and serve.

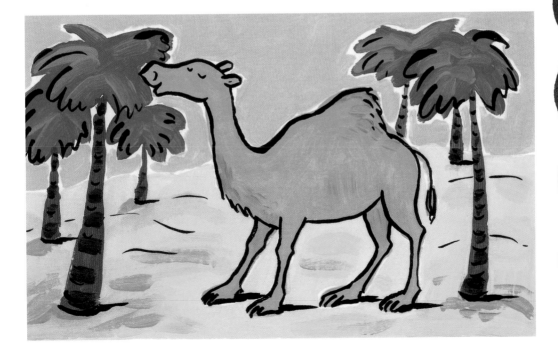

POTATO GRATIN SURPRISE

4–6 SERVINGS

500g/1lb sweet potato, peeled and
    cut into large pieces
500g/1lb potato, peeled and cut
    into large chunks
Generous ¼ tsp each ground
    cinnamon and ground nutmeg
1–2 tbsp unsalted butter
    (optional)
30g/1oz chunk Parmesan cheese,
    finely grated

This can also be turned into potato cakes. Simply blend all the ingredients together and either bake or fry in 1 tbsp olive oil.

Steam both kinds of potato over boiling water until they are tender through, 20–25 minutes.
Preheat the grill, or preheat the oven to 240°C/475°F/Gas 9.
Transfer the potatoes to a large bowl and mash, using a fork so they are of uneven texture. Mix in the spices, with butter if desired, and transfer to a baking dish. Sprinkle the Parmesan cheese over the top.
Grill or bake until the top is crisp and golden and the potatoes are hot through.

CURRIED FISH CHOWDER

4–6 SERVINGS

1 tbsp extra-virgin olive oil
About 3 medium onions , finely
    chopped
250g/8oz potatoes, peeled and
    finely grated
1 carrot, peeled, trimmed and
    finely grated
125ml/4fl oz filtered water
500ml/16fl oz soy milk
½–1 tsp curry powder, to taste
360g/12oz mild white boneless
    fish fillets, cut into 2.5cm/1in
    chunks

TO GARNISH:
Fresh coriander or flat-leaf parsley
Paprika

The soy milk in this recipe makes it a good choice if you're trying to keep dairy to a minimum. Any firm, white fish can be used; salmon is also good.

Heat the oil and onions in a medium, heavy-bottomed frying pan over medium heat. Cover, reduce the heat to medium-low and cook, stirring occasionally, until the onions are turning translucent and have ceased to give off a sharp, hot aroma.
Add the potatoes, carrot and water, stir and bring to a boil. Cook at a simmer until the potatoes and carrots are tender, about 7 minutes.
Add the milk and curry powder, stir, then cover and simmer gently until the flavours have mellowed and the potatoes and carrot have completely cooked, about 30 minutes. You may make the chowder up to this point, then let it sit in the refrigerator overnight to give the flavours a chance to mellow.
Add the fish, stir, then cook until it is opaque through, about 5 minutes. Garnish with coriander or parsley and paprika and serve.

Pizza ideas
• • • • • • • • • • • • •

THIS IS THE IDEAL "FAST FOOD" FOR children as pizza can be assembled in minutes from whatever ingredients you have to hand. Pizza is also an good way to offer vegetables that might otherwise be refused.

The most obvious bases are crusty Italian-style breads, split muffins, wholewheat pitta bread or ready-made wholewheat pizza bases from health food shops. If your child is avoiding wheat, investigate the possibility of making dough from wheat-free flour, from health-food shops or even some supermarkets (see page 186 for mail-order addresses). Grilled polenta slices (*see page 150*) are another ideal wheat-free alternative.

These pizza bases can be served in large portions, or use a small round biscuit cutter to stamp out little circles, perfect for little fingers. Older children also love to help with the preparation – simply do all the chopping and slicing first, then let them help spread the sauce and sprinkle over the toppings.

Cubes of tomato sauce from the freezer are perfect as a sauce base, but shop-bought sauces will do the trick just as well. The topping ideas are as limitless as your cupboard, but here are a few suggestions to get you going, to use alone or in combination. You can also use any of the pasta sauces on pages 160-63.

Despite our conditioning, pizzas do not have to have cheese on them, but if you want to add cheese, choose from the healthy options listed below.

Once you have assembled your pizza, simply bake in a hot oven until the edges of the crusts are just golden and the toppings are cooked through.

- Finely chopped onions
- Sliced mushrooms and peppers
- Courgette and olive slices
- Goat's cheese, crumbled or grated
- Tuna
- Grated carrots
- Thinly sliced marinated artichoke hearts

- Chopped spinach and feta cheese with oregano
- Thinly sliced red onion and minced garlic
- Thinly sliced broccoli florets
- Peas
- Steamed aubergine slices
- Capers
- Thinly sliced fennel and leek

- Sliced aspargus
- Ratatouille
- Sliced soya cheese
- Grated Parmesan (in moderation)
- Pesto sauce
- Cooked minced chicken
- Sardines
- Buffalo milk mozzarella
- Salmon

Simple Asian Rice

This is a meal in itself but if you're pressed for time it is just as successful without the omelette.

4–6 SERVINGS

FOR THE OMELETTE:
2 medium eggs
½ tsp tamari
1 large handful fresh chives
1 tsp sesame oil

FOR THE RICE:
1 tsp sesame oil
225g/7½oz cooked brown rice
60g/2oz fresh or frozen peas
125–185ml/4–6fl oz water
125g/4oz peeled cooked prawns, diced (optional)
Tamari, to serve (optional)
Fresh chopped coriander, to serve

Make the omelette: in a medium bowl, whisk together the eggs, and tamari. Finely chop the chives and whisk them into the egg mixture.

Heat the oil in a non-stick frying pan over medium heat. When the oil is hot, add the egg mixture and cook until it is nearly cooked through, about 2 minutes. Cover, then cook until the top is set. Turn the omelette out onto a work surface and cut into small squares. Set aside.

Make the rice: in the same pan, heat the oil. Add the rice, stir, then add the peas and water. Cook, stirring, until the mixture is hot and the peas are nearly cooked, about 5 minutes. Add the prawns if desired, and cook, stirring, until they are hot through. To serve, stir in the pieces of omelette, season with tamari if desired, and garnish with coriander.

Middle Eastern Rice

Leftover rice in the fridge can be turned into a feast for the family.

4 SERVINGS

2 tbsp extra-virgin olive oil
1 medium onion, finely chopped
2 garlic cloves, finely chopped
2 bay leaves
4 whole cloves
½ tsp ground cinnamon
¼ tsp ground coriander
¼ tsp ground ginger
¼ tsp turmeric
1 small, ripe tomato, peeled and diced
1 small potato, peeled and diced
4 tbsp Herb Stock (see page 176)
225g/7½oz cooked brown rice
1 tsp unsulphured molasses (optional)
¼–½ tsp ground nutmeg

Heat the oil in a large, heavy-bottomed frying pan over medium-high heat. Add the onion, garlic, bay leaves and cloves, stir, then cook until the onion is beginning to turn translucent, about 5 minutes.

Add the spices, stir, then add the tomato, potato and broth. Stir well and bring the broth to a boil, then reduce the heat to medium-low so the broth is simmering. Cover and cook, stirring occasionally, until the potato is tender, 10–15 minutes.

Remove from the heat and stir in the rice. If the mixture tastes slightly acidic from the tomatoes, stir in the molasses. Season with nutmeg to taste, and serve.

Rice ideas
• • • • • • • • • • •

BROWN RICE IS THE IDEAL FAMILY MEAL standby. It is one of the Wonder Foods (*see page 76*), it can easily be prepared in advance and frozen, and it is economical. The recipes on this page are just a few of the ways that you can use rice as a meal base. The most ideal combination is probably a little bit of all the vegetables you have in the refrigerator, perhaps with a bit of tomato sauce or herb stock (*see Recipe Index*) to moisten the mixture and a handful of chopped fresh herbs as a finishing touch. Here are a few more ideas. You can also use any of the pasta sauces on pages 160–63.

• Sliced sautéed onion, celery and grated carrot

• Cannelini beans, chopped fresh basil, tomato sauce and grated Parmesan

• Minced sautéed chicken, onion and grated apple

• Chopped spinach and sautéed onions (with pine kernels for older children)

• Diced sautéed courgette and tomatoes with pesto

• Salmon, peas, chopped bean sprouts and soya sauce

• Diced sautéed peppers and mushrooms

• Chickpeas and diced onions cooked in curry paste with coconut milk

• Kidney beans, sweetcorn kernels, diced tomatoes, chopped spring onions, a sprinkling of ground cumin, a squeeze of lime juice and chopped fresh coriander

• Peas and grated Parmesan

• Sardines in tomato sauce with sautéed onion

• Sautéed sliced leeks, cabbage and mushrooms

MEDITERRANEAN RICE
• •

4–6 SERVINGS

1 small aubergine (250g/8oz), trimmed and diced
1 good-sized courgette (300g/10oz), trimmed and diced
1 medium onion (150g/5oz), diced
1 red pepper, cored, seeded and diced
2 garlic cloves, finely chopped
125ml/4fl oz filtered water
225g/7½oz cooked brown rice

This is a colourful dish that delivers a wide range of nutrients by virtue of the fact that it is colourful (see page 116).

Place the vegetables and water in a frying pan over medium heat. Cover and cook, stirring occasionally, until the vegetables are soft and tender and the flavours have blended, about 1 hour. To serve, either mix with or serve atop brown rice.

MUSHROOM TORTILLA
• •

4 SERVINGS

2 tbsp extra-virgin olive oil
1 shallot, finely chopped
360g/12oz mushrooms, trimmed,
* brushed clean and finely*
chopped
Small handful chopped fresh flat-
* leaf parsley*
5 whole eggs

This is perfect for lunch or breakfast. Serve it in small bite-size pieces
for finger food fans.

Heat half the oil in a large, heavy-bottomed frying pan over
medium heat. Add the shallot and cook, stirring often, until it is
transparent and tender, about 3 minutes. Add the mushrooms
and stir, then cook, stirring often, until tender, about 8 minutes.
Finely chop the parsley, add it to the mushrooms and stir. Cook
until the flavour of the parsley has mellowed, an additional 2
minutes, then remove from the heat and set aside.
In a 23cm/9in frying pan, heat the remaining oil over medium
heat until it is hot but not smoking.
Whisk the eggs until they are just broken and combined, but not
so much that they become fluffy. Stir the mushrooms into the
eggs, then pour the mixture into the frying pan and stir once or
twice. Let cook until the bottom is set and bubbles come up
through the top of the egg, which is still liquid, 2–3 minutes.
Preheat the grill.
Place the pan about 12.5cm/5in from the grill and cook just until
the top of the tortilla is set, about 1 minute. Do not overcook – the
tortilla should be tender and moist, and not the least bit hard.
Serve hot or cold.

BEAN & GARLIC STEW
• •

4–6 SERVINGS

250g/8oz dried borlotti or other
* beans*
3 garlic cloves, peeled
1 bay leaf
17g/6oz Swiss chard, rinsed,
* trimmed and diced*

TO GARNISH:
2 garlic cloves, finely chopped
4tbsp extra-virgin olive oil

You can substitute fresh or frozen spinach for the Swiss chard. Canned
beans in unsalted water can also be used if you're pressed for time.

Place the beans in a large saucepan and cover them with 5cm/2in
water. Bring to a boil, covered, over high heat. Remove from the
heat and let sit for 1 hour.
Drain the beans and cover them with fresh cold water. Add the
whole garlic cloves, the bay leaf and onion. Cover and bring to a
boil, then reduce the heat so the liquid is simmering merrily.
Cook until the beans are tender, about 1 hour. Check occasionally
to be sure there is enough water to cover the beans.
Add the chard to the beans, cover and cook until the chard is
tender through, 20–30 minutes.
Make the garnish in a small pan by heating the garlic with the oil
over low heat, just until the garlic begins to turn golden, about 10
minutes. Remove from the heat and transfer to a small serving
bowl. Keep warm.
Ladle stew into bowls and pass the garlic and oil alongside.

TUNA WITH TWENTY GARLIC CLOVES

Serve this with oven-roasted potatoes for a delicious family meal.

4 SERVINGS

2 tbsp olive oil
20 garlic cloves, with skin
250ml/8fl oz Herb Stock (see page 176) or dry white wine
4 medium tuna steaks
Finely chopped fresh flat-leaf parsley, to garnish

In a large, heavy-bottomed frying pan, heat the oil and garlic cloves over medium heat. Stir, cover and cook, stirring occasionally, until the garlic begins to soften, about 10 minutes. Slowly add the broth, stir and gently scrape up any brown bits from the bottom of the pan. Cook, partially covered, until the liquid has reduced by about one-quarter, about 4 minutes. Rinse and pat dry the tuna steaks and add them to the pan. Partially cover and cook until the tuna is opaque through, 10–12 minutes. Transfer the tuna to a warmed serving platter. Increase the heat under the pan and cook the juices, stirring, until they have reduced by half, about 4 minutes. Pour the juices and garlic over the tuna, garnish with parsley and serve. Before serving to children, remove the skin from the tuna and ensure there are no bones. To extract the garlic, simply press on the clove and the purée will emerge. Spread this atop the tuna, or eat it alongside.

AROMATIC GREEN BEANS

Instead of the oil and herb dressing used here, you could use half the quantity of Wonderful Walnut Pesto given on page 162.

4 SERVINGS

500g/1lb fine green beans, trimmed and cut in bite-size lengths
3 tbsp extra-virgin olive oil or walnut oil
Mixture of fresh herbs, including savory, thyme and basil

Steam the green beans until tender so they can be chewed by little teeth, 5-8 minutes.
While the beans are cooking, blend the olive oil and herbs in a large serving bowl.
When the beans are cooked, add immediately to the dressing and toss well. Serve at room temperature.

GHEE
••••••••

MAKES 375ML/12FL OZ

500g/1lb unsalted butter

There are quicker ways of making ghee, but slow cooking ensures that the butter and milk solids do not burn, which is healthier.

Preheat the oven to 110°C/225°F/Gas ¼.
Place the butter in an ovenproof saucepan large enough to hold it with plenty of room to spare. Cook the butter in the oven until it has fully melted, the solids have floated to the top and the milky substance at the bottom of the pan is golden, 1½ hours.
Remove from the heat and strain the solids from the top. Pour the pure yellow, melted butter (the ghee) off the milky substance in the bottom of the pan. Discard the solids and the milky substance that is left. Store the ghee in the refrigerator in an airtight container. It will keep for several months.

HERB STOCK
••••••••••••••••••••

MAKES ABOUT
1.25 LITRES/2 PINTS

5cm/4in sprig fresh rosemary
2 bay leaves
15 sprigs fresh thyme
10 sage leaves
2 garlic cloves
1 onion, quartered
1.5 litres/2½ pints water

Freeze this in ice-cube trays for individual serving-size portions.

Place all the ingredients in a stock pot, cover and bring to a boil over medium-high heat. Reduce the heat so the liquid just simmers, then simmer for about 20 minutes.
Remove from the heat and strain. Use the stock immediately or freeze.

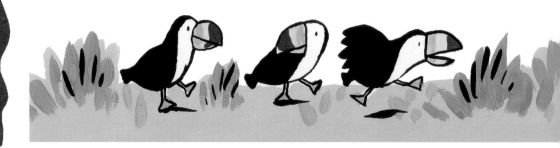

YOGHURT CURRY DRESSING

MAKES 250ML/8FL OZ

250ml/8fl oz plain yoghurt
1 tsp curry powder

This is a simple idea that peps up all kinds of dishes. Add to salads, meat and fish dishes or baked potatoes. It also accompanies rice dishes very well.

Whisk together the yoghurt and curry powder. Refrigerate in an airtight container for up to 1 week.

TERRIFIC TUNA SAUCE

MAKES ABOUT
375ML/12FL OZ

300g/10oz canned albacore tuna,
    packed in oil or brine, drained
60g/2oz capers, drained
6 tbsp extra-virgin olive oil

Serve as a dipping sauce with vegetable sticks, crackers or bread.

Place the tuna and capers in a food processor and process. With the machine running, add the oil in a thin stream and continue processing until the mixture has turned an ivory colour and is quite smooth and light, about 8 minutes.

SAUCY AVOCADO

MAKES ABOUT 250ML/8FL OZ

2 avocados, peeled, stoned and
    coarsely chopped
2 tbsp freshly squeezed lemon juice
1 garlic clove, diced
1 tbsp extra-virgin olive oil
¼ tsp ground cumin

Serve as a spread on bread, or as a dip with raw vegetables. It is also good as a salad dressing, diluted with a little plain yoghurt if necessary.

Place all the ingredients in a food processor and blend until very smooth.

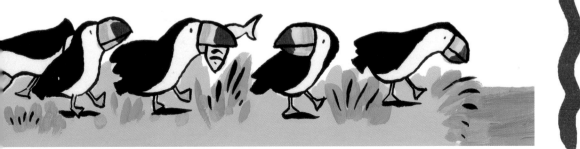

DATE OAT WEDGES

MAKES ONE 23CM/9IN CAKE
(UP TO 12 WEDGES)

3 whole eggs
1 tsp unsulphured molasses
1 tsp vanilla extract
90g/3oz oat flour
1 tsp baking powder
3 tbsp rolled oats
200g/7oz chopped dates
2 tsp grated orange zest

If you can't find oat flour, simply place oats in a food processor and process them until they make a fairly fine flour.

Preheat the oven to 190°C/375°F/Gas 5. Butter and flour a 23cm/9in cake tin.
In a large bowl or the bowl of an electric mixer, whisk the eggs with the molasses and vanilla extract until they are light and fluffy. Mix in the oat flour, baking powder and 2 tbsp of the oats. Fold in the dates and orange zest and turn the batter into the prepared tin. Sprinkle the remaining oats on top.
Bake in the middle of the oven until the cake springs back when touched, about 20 minutes. Remove from the oven and let cool on a wire rack. Cut into wedges to serve.

CORNMEAL GINGER COOKIES

MAKES ABOUT 55

190g/6½oz fine cornmeal
30g/1oz instant milk powder
2 tsp baking powder
½ tsp ground nutmeg
½ tsp ground ginger
70g/2½oz rolled oats
4 tbsp mild vegetable oil or melted,
    unsalted butter
125ml/4fl oz unsulphured
    molasses
4 tbsp honey
1 egg
4 tbsp milk
60g/2oz raisins, chopped

Have these to hand to offer instead of the usual shop bought biscuits – don't bring out too many though because they will all go very quickly!

Preheat the oven to 180°C/350°F/Gas 4. Line 2 baking sheets with parchment paper.
In a medium bowl, mix together all the dry ingredients.
In another medium bowl, whisk together the oil, molasses, honey, egg and milk until well blended. Stir in the dry ingredients and mix until just blended, then stir in the raisins.
Drop the batter by teaspoonfuls onto the prepared baking sheets. Bake in the middle of the oven until the cookies are puffed and spring back when touched, about 10 minutes. Remove from the baking sheets and let cool on a wire rack.

INDIAN PUDDING

6 SERVINGS

This is a traditional early American recipe.

1 litre/1¾ pints milk
55g/scant 2oz coarse cornmeal
185ml/6fl oz unsulphured
  molasses
125g/4oz unsalted butter
1 tsp ground ginger
½ tsp ground cinnamon
Pinch ground cloves
70g/2½oz raisins
Plain yoghurt, to serve (optional)

Preheat the oven to 180°C/350°F/Gas 4. Butter a 1.5 litre/2¾ pint soufflé dish or mould.

Scald the milk in a large saucepan over medium heat. When the milk is scalded, whisk in the cornmeal and cook, stirring frequently, until the mixture thickens, about 15 minutes. Whisk in the molasses, remove from the heat, then stir in the butter, spices and raisins.

Pour the mixture into the prepared dish and bake in the middle of the oven until the pudding is cooked through, 1½ hours.

Remove the pudding from the oven and let cool until no longer scalding. Serve with yoghurt alongside, if desired.

CREAMY FRUIT PUDDING

4–6 SERVINGS

You can stir any fruit you like into this pudding, particularly fresh berries.

1 whole banana
1 tsp freshly squeezed lemon juice
1 litre/1¾ pints fruit juice
  (e.g. apple, strawberry, cherry
  or grape)
6 tbsp (55g/scant 2oz) rice flour
Plain yoghurt, to garnish
  (optional)

Peel and dice the banana and place it in the bottom of a 1.5 litre/2¾ pint soufflé dish or mould. Pour the lemon juice over the banana to keep it from browning.

Bring the fruit juice to a boil in a medium saucepan over medium-high heat. Whisk the rice flour into the juice, return the mixture to the boil and continue cooking until it has thickened substantially, 8–10 minutes. Remove from the heat, then pour over the banana in the dish. Let cool to room temperature, and serve with yoghurt alongside if desired. This may be eaten warm, or chilled in the refrigerator and eaten cold.

CHOCOLATE PUDDING

6 SERVINGS

Try to use chocolate with 70% cocoa solids and organic is even better.

3tbsp cornflour
1tbsp tapioca
500ml/16fl oz milk
75ml/3fl oz honey
60g/2oz unsweetened chocolate
1tsp vanilla extract

In a saucepan, mix the cornflour, tapioca and milk over medium heat. Add the honey and chocolate and cook, stirring frequently, until the mixture thickens. Do not let it boil.
Just before removing the pudding from the heat, stir in the vanilla extract. Pour into a dish, let cool to room temperature, then refrigerate until chilled.

APPLE-POLENTA COBBLER

4–6 SERVINGS

This is simple, delicious and sure to become a family favourite.

2 large apples, peeled, cored and
*   cut into very thin slices*
¼tsp ground cinnamon
2 eggs, separated
4tbsp honey
4tbsp molasses
250ml/8fl oz milk
250g/8oz fine polenta
200g/7oz wholewheat flour
1tbsp baking powder

Preheat the oven to 200°C/400°F/Gas 6. Place the apples in the bottom of a baking dish so they are about 2.5cm/1in deep. Sprinkle the apples with the cinnamon.
In a small bowl, whisk together the egg yolks, honey, molasses and milk. Measure the dry ingredients into a large bowl and mix them. Add the wet ingredients and stir quickly, just until they are blended.
Whisk the egg whites until they hold soft peaks, then fold into the batter. Pour the batter over the apples and bake until the batter is puffed and springs back when touched, about 30 minutes.

Tropical Fruit Salad

This is the ideal dessert for children – it is colourful, delicious and so good for them. This recipe is just a blueprint experiment with different fruit, according to the season and your child's tastes. Toss together the following ingredients: 1 mango, peeled, stoned and cut into tiny dice; flesh from ½ small cantaloupe melon, cut into tiny dice; 1 kiwi, peeled and cut into tiny dice; 70g/2½ oz raspberries; 5 dates, stoned and cut into tiny dice; 1 tbsp freshly squeezed lime juice and serve immediately.

WHOLEWHEAT FRUIT SHORTCAKE

6 SERVINGS

Older children will enjoy making the shortcakes with you.

250g/8oz wholewheat flour
2½tsp baking powder
½tsp freshly grated nutmeg
3-6 tsp unsalted butter
125-185ml/4-6fl oz milk
400g/14oz fresh or frozen and
    thawed mixed red berries
Live plain yoghurt

Preheat the oven to 220°C/425°F/Gas 7.
Place the flour and baking powder in a bowl and mix together.
Using your fingertips or a pastry cutter, blend in the butter until it
is the size of very small peas and blended with the flour. With a
fork, stir in enough milk to make a moist but not wet dough.
Pat out the dough to an 18cm/7½in square, then cut the square
into 6 equal pieces. Bake in the middle of the oven until the
shortcakes are puffed and slightly golden, about 25 minutes.
Remove from the oven, cut the shortcakes in half horizontally
(through their thickness) and place the bottom piece of each on a
plate. Top each with berries and a dollop of yoghurt, then
balance the top pieces of shortcake atop the berries.

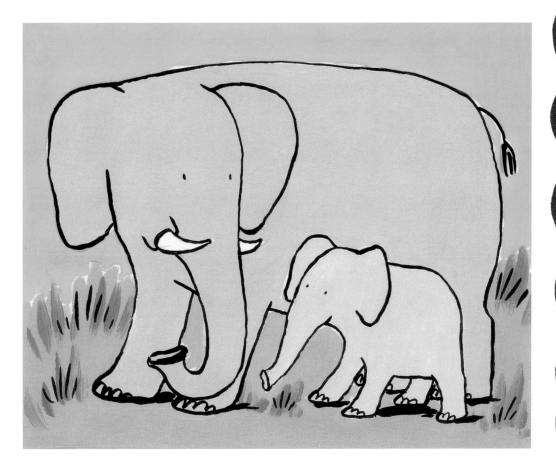

CHICKEN NIBBLES

• •

4–6 SERVINGS

125ml/4fl oz live yoghurt
250–375g/8–12oz chicken
(preferably dark meat) without
skin
150g/5oz raw almonds
75g/2½oz flour
2–3 tbsp extra-virgin olive oil

The almonds make these a healthier option then the supermarket variety.
Leftovers can be frozen.

Place the yoghurt in a medium, shallow bowl. Cut the chicken
into thin strips, add them to the yoghurt and stir so they are
coated.

Place the almonds in a food processor and blend until they are
finely ground (but not so long that they turn into a paste). Add
the flour and blend until the almonds and the flour are evenly
mixed.

Preheat the oven to 230°C/450°F/Gas 9. Place 2 tbsp of the oil in
a large, heavy roasting tin or skillet and place in the hot oven
until the oil is hot but not smoking.

Dredge the chicken pieces in the almond and flour mixture so
they are completely coated, then place them in one layer in the
tin with the hot oil, making sure not to crowd the tin (you may
need to cook the chicken in 2 batches, and you may want to add
the additional oil). Cook until the chicken is golden on one side,
about 3 minutes. Turn and cook until the chicken is cooked
through and golden on the other side, an additional 2 minutes.
Repeat with any remaining chicken.

Transfer the chicken to a plate and serve it when it is cool enough
to handle, with additional yoghurt as a dipping sauce, if desired.

FISH FINGERS

• • • • • • • • • • • • • • • • • • •

4–6 SERVINGS

75g/2½oz almonds, ground not
too fine
½ tsp dried oregano
250g/8oz fresh tuna, mackerel or
swordfish, skin and bones
removed, cut into 5 × 1.25cm/
2 × ½in pieces
2–3 tbsp extra-virgin olive oil

You may also use any white fish in the cod family.

In a small bowl, mix together the almonds and oregano. Transfer
them to a plate, shallow bowl or the work surface.

Rinse the fish and leave the pieces damp. Roll the fish in the
almond mixture, pressing it into the fish.

Heat the oil in a frying pan over medium-high heat. When it is
hot, sauté the fish until it is golden and opaque through and the
almonds are toasty. This will take 1–4 minutes per side,
depending on the fish.

Transfer to a serving dish and let little fingers go!

TEMPURA VEGETABLES

4–6 SERVINGS

Even the most reluctant of vegetable eaters will not be able to resist this.

1kg/2lb mixed vegetables
  (e.g. courgettes, potatoes, sweet
  potatoes, broccoli)
90g/3oz flour
250ml/8fl oz sparkling mineral
  water
500ml/16fl oz mild oil such as
  safflower or sunflower
375ml/12fl oz extra-virgin olive oil

Trim and peel the vegetables, if necessary, then rinse them and pat them dry. Cut the potatoes into very thin slices. Separate the broccoli florets into small pieces, and slice the broccoli stalks very thinly.

Place the flour in a large bowl and whisk in the sparkling water. Line a baking sheet with several layers of unprinted brown paper, or with paper towels.

Heat the oils in an electric deep-fat fryer until they are hot but not smoking. When the oil is ready, dip several pieces of vegetable into the batter, letting any excess drip off. Using tongs, place enough vegetables in the pan so they float in an even layer on the surface without crowding each other. Cook until they are golden, 1 minute or less. Remove from the oil, let drain, and set on the paper-covered baking sheet until they are cool enough to handle. Serve.

SALMON DUMPLINGS

4–6 SERVINGS

These are also good served on top of a bed of steamed spinach seasoned with fresh lemon juice.

500g/1lb salmon fillet, skinned,
  rinsed and cut into chunks
1 large egg
1 small handful fresh flat-leaf
  parsley
1 small bunch chives

Place the salmon in a food processor and blend until homogeneous. Add the egg and blend until smooth. Chop the parsley and chives, add to the salmon and egg and blend once or twice, just until incorporated.

Bring a medium saucepan of water to a boil. Using 2 teaspoons, form the salmon mixture into small balls and drop them into the boiling water without crowding the pan. Let them cook until they are pale pink through and rise to the surface of the water, about 3 minutes. Remove from the water with a slotted spoon, let drain, then arrange on a platter. Serve when they are cool enough to handle.

USEFUL
REFERENCES

This list is intended to help you begin finding out more information about areas of childcare and nutrition that may interest you. It is not intended as a comprehensive list, nor does inclusion imply any warranty for the organizations' services.

ALLERGY ASSOCIATIONS AND SUPPLIERS

Allergy Free Direct
Mail order foods
www.allergyfreedirect.co.uk
01865 722003

Allergy UK
Leading medical charity
www.allergyuk.org
Helpline: 020 8303 8583

Anaphylaxis Campaign
www.anaphylaxis.org.uk
01252 542029

The Healthy House
For allergy-free bedding and other supplies
www.healthy-house.co.uk
01453 752216

Stamp Collection/ Buxton Foods
Gluten and dairy-free products
www.stamp-collection.co.uk
020 7637 5505

Cooking Without
Allergy-free cooking
Barbara Cousins, Thorsons, 2000

(See also Organix Baby Foods below)

BABY FOODS

Beech-Nut Stages
Beech-Nut Nutrition.Corp., Canajoharie,
NY 13317, USA

Cow & Gate Organic Choice
www.cowandgate.co.uk
08457 623623

Hipp Organic
www.hipp.co.uk
0845 0501351

Mothers Recipe Organic
Produced and stocked by Boots the Chemist

Organix Baby Foods
Firs baby food company to receive the 'free from' award from Allergy UK the leading medical charity for their baby foods and cereals.
www.babyorganix.co.uk
0800 393511

BREAST-FEEDING

La Leche League (Great Britain)
www.laleche.org.uk
020 7242 1278

National Childbirth Trust
Breast feeding counsellors and mothers' groups
www.nct-online.org.uk
0870 444 8707

Breast is Best
Penny and Andrew Stanway, Pan Books 1978
(revised 1996)

CHILD BEHAVIOUR

Food Fights
David Haslam, Hutchinson, 1986
(revised 1995)

Food: Too Faddy? Too Fat?
John Pearce, Thorsons, 1991

(See also Learning Difficulties)

FOOD ADDITIVES

Foresight
Pre-conceptual care –
 also information on food additives
www.foresight-preconception.org.uk
01483 427839

E for Additives
Maurice Hanssen, Thorsons, 1984
(revised 1988)

The Food Magazine
Published by The Food Commission, an
independent watchdog. Encompasses The
Parent Jury which seeks to improve the quality
of children's foods and drinks.
www.foodcomm.org.uk
www.parentsjury.org
020 7837.2250

The Food Our Children Eat
Joanna Blythman, Fourth Estate, 2000

FORMULA MILKS

Babynat Organic Infant Formula Milk
Info@organico.co.uk
0118 951 0518

Nanny Goat Infant Formula Milk
Suitable for all infants, particularly those with
cow's milk sensitivity
www.vitacare.co.uk
Helpline: 0800 328 5826

Omenocomfort
A milk specifically designed to ease digestive and
colic problems. It does this with partially
hydrolysed (pre-digested) proteins, reduced
lactose and the addition of prebiotic
oligosaccharides. Also contains some essential
fatty acids. Made by Cow & Gate.
www.cowandgate.co.uk
Careline: 08457 623624

LCP supplemented formulas
The following milks contain the two important
LCPs (long-chain polyunsaturated fatty acids)
for brain, nervous and eye development
(DHA and AA):

Cow & Gate range:
Nutriprem 1 Low Birthweight Formula (hospital
use only)
Nutriprem 2 Special Infant Milk (for low
birthweight infants prior to and once discharged
from hospital).
Premium (whey dominant first infant milk)
www.cowandgate.co.uk
Careline: 08457 623623

Milupa range:
Pre-Aptamil (for low birthweight infants
in neonatal units)
Aptamil First (whey dominant first infant milk)
Aptamil Extra (casein dominant milk – currently
the only milk for hungrier bottlefed babies
on the UK market which contains LCPs)
www.milupa.co.uk
Careline: 08457 623 628

LEARNING DIFFICULTIES

The Hyperactive Children's Support Group
Send an SAE for a list of information
leaflets to order, or free online.
71 Whyke Lane, Chichester,
West Sussex PO19 2LD
www.hacsg.org.uk

The LCP Solution
Jacqueline Stordy, Macmillan, 2002

Effalex
This is the essential fatty acid
supplement used in research into
children with learning difficulties.
Nutricia Helpline: 0870 750 4526

NUTRITIONAL SUPPLEMENTS, SUPPLIERS OF

Biocare
Mail order available; excellent range of
products for babies and small
children incluing banana fort powder, bifidum
infantis bacteria powder and
liquid vitamin and mineral drops.
www.biocare.co.uk
0121 433 3727

The Health and Diet Company
Stocks FSC and other products, several outlets.
www.gnc.co.uk
0845 076 5358

GNC
A wide range of products, several
outlets and mail order.
www.gnc.co.uk
0845 601 3248

Higher Nature
Mail order available. Suppliers of flax oil
and essential balance oil in addition
to many other products.
www.highernature.co.uk
01435 882880

Nature's Best (Lamberts)
Mail order available.
www.naturesbestonline.com
01892 552117

The Nutri Centre
Full range of products. Flora Oils (Udo's Blend
Oil) and green clay also available.
Mail order available.7 Park Crescent, London
W1N 3HE (and other outlets)
www.nutricentre.com
020 7436 5122

Quest Vitamins
Available at Holland & Barrett
www.questvitamins.co.uk
0121 359 0056

Revital
A comprehensive range of products.
Several outlets and mail order.
www.revital.com
0800 252875

Solgar
www.solgar.com
01442 890355

Viridian
A company with a strong ecological/ethical
approach
www.viridian-nutrition.com
01327 878050

NUTRITIONAL THERAPISTS, REGISTERS

British Association for Nutritional Therapists (BANT)
www.bant.org.uk

British Society for Allergy, Environmental and Nutritional Medicine (BSAENM)
For a list of medical doctors who
practice nutritional medicine
www.bsaenm.org
0906 302 0010

The Institute for Optimum Nutrition (ION)
www.ion.ac.uk
020 8877 9993

ORGANIC/SPECIALITY FOOD SUPPLIERS

Soil Association
Directory of local organic suppliers,
box schemes, home delivery
and collection points
www.soilassociation.org/SA/directory.nsf/
0117 929 0661

OrganicFood.co.uk
www.organicfood.co.uk
Free online magazine with a wealth of
information about where, why and how
to buy organic foods.

Mail order companies:

The Food Ferry
www.foodferry.com
020 7498 0827

Fresh Food Company
www.freshfood.co.uk
020 8969 0351

Organics Direct
www.organicsdirect.co.uk
01604 791911

Simply Organic
www.simplyorganic.net
0845 1000 444

VACCINATIONS

JABS
www.jabs.org.uk
01942 713565

The Informed Parent
www.informedparent.co.uk
020 8861 1022

VEGETARIANISM

The Vegetarian Society
www.vegsoc.org

RECIPE INDEX

INDEX